Springer Series in Statistics

Advisors:
S. Fienberg, J. Gani, K. Krickeberg,
I. Olkin, B. Singer, N. Wermuth

Springer Series in Statistics

(continued after index)

Phillip Good

Permutation Tests

A Practical Guide to Resampling Methods for Testing Hypotheses

With 13 Illustrations

Springer-Verlag
New York Berlin Heidelberg London Paris
Tokyo Hong Kong Barcelona Budapest

Phillip Good
West Coast University
440 Shatto Place
Los Angeles, CA 90020-1765
USA

Cover illustration: Building a minimal spanning tree.

Library of Congress Cataloging-in-Publication Data
Good, Phillip I.
    Permutation tests: a practical guide to resampling methods for
testing hypotheses/Phillip Good.
        p.   cm.—(Springer series in statistics)
    Includes bibliographical references and index.
    ISBN 0-387-94097-9
    1. Statistical hypothesis testing.   2. Resampling (Statistics)
I. Title.   II. Series.
QA277.G643   1993
519.5′6—dc20   93-9062

Printed on acid-free paper.

Production managed by Natalie Johnson; manufacturing supervised by Jacqui Ashri·
Typeset by Asco Trade Typesetting Ltd., Hong Kong·
Printed and bound by Edwards Brothers, Inc., Ann Arbor, MI.
Printed in the United States of America.

9 8 7 6 5 4 3 2 1

ISBN 0-387-94097-9 Springer-Verlag New York Berlin Heidelberg
ISBN 3-540-94097-9 Springer-Verlag Berlin Heidelberg New York

Preface

Permutation tests permit us to choose the test statistic best suited to the task at hand. This freedom of choice opens up a thousand practical applications, including many which are beyond the reach of conventional parametric statistics. Flexible, robust in the face of missing data and violations of assumptions, the permutation test is among the most powerful of statistical procedures. Through sample size reduction, permutation tests can reduce the costs of experiments and surveys.

This text on the application of permutation tests in biology, medicine, science, and engineering may be used as a step-by-step self-guiding reference manual by research workers and as an intermediate text for undergraduates and graduates in statistics and the applied sciences with a first course in statistics and probability under their belts.

Research workers in the applied sciences are advised to read through Chapters 1 and 2 once quickly before proceeding to Chapters 3 through 8 which cover the principal applications they are likely to encounter in practice.

Chapter 9 is a must for the practitioner, with advice for coping with real-life emergencies such as missing or censored data, after-the-fact covariates, and outliers.

Chapter 10 uses practical applications in archeology, biology, climatology, education and social science to show the research worker how to develop new permutation statistics to meet the needs of specific applications. The practitioner will find Chapter 10 a source of inspiration as well as a practical guide to the development of new and novel statistics.

The expert system in Chapter 11 will guide you to the correct statistic for your application. Chapter 12, more "must" reading, provides practical advice on experimental design and shows how to document the results of permutation tests for publication.

Chapter 13 describes techniques for reducing computation time; and a guide to off-the-shelf statistical software is provided in an appendix.

The sequence of recommended readings is somewhat different for the student and will depend on whether he or she is studying the permutation tests by themselves or as part of a larger course on resampling methods encompassing both the permutation test and the bootstrap resampling method.

This book can replace a senior-level text on testing hypotheses. I have also found it of value in introducing students who are primarily mathematicians to the applications which make statistics a unique mathematical science. Chapters 1, 2, and 14 provide a comprehensive introduction to the theory. Despite its placement in the latter part of the text, Chapter 14, on the theory of permutation tests, is self-standing. Chapter 3 on applications also deserves a careful reading. Here in detail are the basic testing situations and the basic tests to be applied to them. Chapters 4, 5, and 6 may be used to supplement Chapter 3, time permitting (the first part of Chapter 6 describing the Fisher exact test is a must). Rather than skipping from section to section, it might be best for the student to consider one of these latter chapters in depth—supplementing his or her study with original research articles.

My own preference is to parallel discussions of permutation methods with discussion of a second resampling method, the bootstrap. Again, Chapters 1, 2, and 3—supplemented with portions of Chapter 14—are musts. Chapter 7, on tests of dependence, is a natural sequel. Students in statistical computing also are asked to program and test at least one of the advanced algorithms in Chapter 12.

For the reader's convenience, the bibliography is divided into four parts: the first consists of 34 seminal articles; the second of a dozen or so background articles referred to in the text that are not directly concerned with permutation methods; the third of 105 articles on increasing computational efficiency; and a fourth, principal bibliography of over 550 articles and books on the theory and application of permutation techniques.

Exercises are included at the end of each chapter to enhance and reinforce your understanding. But the best exercise of all is to substitute your own data for the examples in the text.

My thanks to Symantek, TSSI, and Perceptronics without whose Grand-View® outliner, Exact® equation generator, and Einstein Writer® word processor this text would not have been possible.

I am deeply indebted to Mike Chernick for our frequent conversations and his many invaluable insights, to Alan Forsythe and Karim Hiriji for reading and commenting on portions of this compuscript and to my instructors at Berkeley including E. Fix, J. Hodges, E. Lehmann, and J. Neyman.

P.G.
Huntington Beach, CA

Contents

CHAPTER 1

A Wide Range of Applications

1.1. Permutation Tests

The chief value of permutation tests lies in their wide range of applications:

Permutation tests can be applied to continuous, ordered and categorical data, and to values that are normal, almost normal, and non-normally distributed.

For almost every parametric and nonparametric test, one may obtain a distribution-free permutation counterpart. The resulting permutation test is usually as powerful as or more powerful than alternative approachs. And permutation methods can sometimes be made to work when other statistical methods fail (see Chapter 3 Section 3.4 and Chapter 10).

Permutation tests can be applied to homogeneous (text book) and to heterogeneous (real life) data when subpopulations are mixed together (see Section 10.3), when covariables must be taken into account (see Sections 4.3, 6.5, and 9.2), and when repeated measures on a single subject must be adjusted for (Section 5.5). The ability of permutation methods to be adapted to real-world situations is what led to my writing this book for the practitioner.

1.1.1. Applications

Permutation tests have been applied in cluster analysis [Hubert and Levin, 1976], Fourier analysis [Friedman and Lane, 1980], multivariate analysis [Arnold, 1964; Mielke, 1986] and single-subject analysis [Kazdin, 1976]; (but see Kazdin [1980]). In anthropology [Fisher, 1936], agriculture [Kempthorne, 1952], archaeology [Berry, Kvamme, and Mielke, 1985], atmospheric science [Adderley, 1961; Tukey, Brillinger, and Jones, 1978], biology [Howard, 1980], botany [Mitchell-Olds, 1986, 1987], ecology [Manly, 1983; Mueller and Altenberg, 1985], education [Manly, 1988], epidemiology [Glass, Mantel, Gunz, and Spears, 1971], genetics [Karlin and Williams, 1984], geography [Royaltey, Astrachen, and Sokal, 1975], geology [Clark,

1989], medicine [Bross, 1964; Feinstein, 1973; McKinney, Young, Hartz Bi-Fong Lee, 1989], molecular biology [Barker and Dayhoff, 1972; Karlin, Ghandour, Ost, Tauare, and Korph, 1983], paleontology [Marcus, 1969], sociology [Marascuilo and McSweeny, 1977] and reliability [Kalbfleisch and Prentice, 1980].

Permutation methods are relatively impervious to complications that defeat other statistical techniques. Outliers and "broad tails" may be defended against through the use of preliminary rank or robust transformations, (Section 9.3). Missing data often is corrected for automatically. Missing and censored data may affect the power of a permutation test, but not its existence or exactness. A most powerful unbiased permutation test often works in cases where a most powerful parametric test fails for lack of knowledge of some yet unknown nuisance parameter [Lehmann, 1986]; [Good 1989, 1991, 1992].

A major reason permutation tests have such a wide range of applications is that they require only one or two relatively weak assumptions, e.g., that the underlying distributions are symmetric, and/or the alternatives are simples shifts in value. The permutation test can even be applied to finite populations (see Section 2.4).

1.2. "I Lost the Labels"

Shortly after I received my doctorate in statistics, I decided that if I really wanted to help bench scientists apply statistics I ought to become a scientist myself. So back to school I went to learn all about physiology and aging in cells raised in petri dishes.

I soon learned there was a great deal more to an experiment than the random assignment of subjects to treatments. In general, 90% of my effort was spent in mastering various arcane laboratory techniques, 9% in developing new techniques to span the gap between what had been done and what I really wanted to do, and a mere 1% on the experiment itself. But the moment of truth came finally—it had to if I were to publish and not perish—and I succeeded in cloning human diploid fibroblasts in eight culture dishes: Four of these dishes were filled with a conventional nutrient solution and four held an experimental "life-extending" solution to which Vitamin E had been added.

I waited three weeks with my fingers crossed—there is always a risk of contamination with cell cultures—but at the end of this test period three dishes of each type had survived. My technician and I transplanted the cells, let them grow for 24 hours in contact with a radioactive label, and then fixed and stained them before covering them with a photographic emulsion.

Ten days passed and we were ready to examine the autoradiographs. Two years had elapsed since I first envisioned this experiment and now the results were in: I had the six numbers I needed.

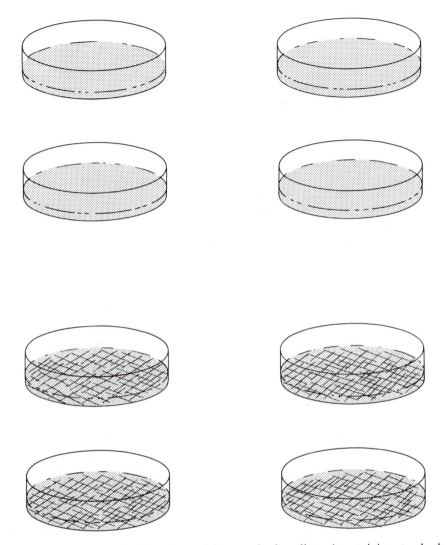

Figure 1.1. Eight petri dishes, 4 containing standard medium, 4 containing standard medium supplemented by Vitamin E. Ten cells innoculated in each dish.

"I've lost the labels," my technician said as he handed me the results.

"What!?" Without the labels, I had no way of knowing which cell cultures had been treated with Vitamin E and which had not.

"121, 118, 110, 34, 12, 22." I read and reread these six numbers over and over again. If the first three counts were from treated colonies and the last three were from untreated, then I had found the fountain of youth. Otherwise, I really had nothing to report.

1.3. Five Steps to a Permutation Test

How had I reached that conclusion?

In succeeding chapters, you will learn to apply permutation techniques to a wide variety of testing problems ranging from the simple to the complex. In each case, you will follow the same five-step procedure that we follow in this example:

1. Analyze the problem.
2. Choose a test statistic.
3. Compute the test statistic for the original labelling of the observations.
4. Rearrange (permute) the labels and recompute the test statistic for the rearranged labels. Repeat until you obtain the distribution of the test statistic for all possible permutations.
5. Accept or reject the hypothesis using this permutation distribution as a guide.

1.3.1. Analyze the Problem

Let's take a second, more formal look at the problem of the missing labels. First, we identify the hypothesis and alternative of interest:

I wanted to assess the life-extending properties of a new experimental treatment. To do this, I divided my cell cultures into two groups: one grown in a standard medium and one grown in a medium containing Vitamin E. At the conclusion of the experiment and after the elimination of several contaminated cultures, both groups consisted of three independently treated dishes.

My null hypothesis is that the growth potential of a culture will not be affected by the presence of Vitamin E in the media. The alternative of interest is that cells grown in the presence of Vitamin E would be capable of many more cell divisions.

Under the null hypothesis, the labels "treated" and "untreated" provide no information about the outcomes, as the observations are expected to have more or less the same values in each of the two experimental groups. I am free to exchange the labels.

1.3.2. Choose a Test Statistic

The next step in the permutation method is to choose a test statistic that discriminates between the hypothesis and the alternative. The statistic I chose was the sum of the counts in the group that had been treated with Vitamin E. If the alternative is true this sum ought to be larger than the sum of the observations in the untreated group. If the null hypothesis is true, that is, if it doesn't make any difference which treatment the cells receive, then the sums of the two groups of observations should be approximately the same. One sum might be smaller or larger than the other by chance, but the two shouldn't be all that different.

1.3.3. Compute the Test Statistic

The third step in the permutation method is to compute the test statistic for each of the possible relabellings. But to compute the test statistic for the data as it had been labelled originally, I had to find the labels! Fortunately, I had kept a record of the treatments independent of my technician. In fact, I had deliberately not let my technician know which cultures were which in order to ensure he would give them equal care in handling. As it happened, the first three observations he showed me—121, 118, and 110 were those belonging to the cultures that had received Vitamin E. The value of the test statistic for the observations as originally labelled is 349: 121 + 118 + 110.

1.3.4. Rearrange the Observations

We now rearrange or permute the observations, randomly reassigning the six labels, three "treated" and three "untreated," to the six observations: for example, treated, 121 118 34, and untreated, 110 12 22. In this rearrangement,

	First Group			Second Group			Sum_1
1.	121	118	110	34	22	12	349
2.	121	118	34	110	22	12	273
3.	121	110	34	118	22	12	265
4.	118	110	34	121	22	12	262
5.	121	118	22	110	34	12	261
6.	121	110	22	118	34	12	253
7.	121	118	12	110	34	22	251
8.	118	110	22	121	34	12	250
9.	121	110	12	118	34	22	243
10.	118	110	12	121	34	22	240
11.	121	34	22	118	110	12	177
12.	118	34	22	121	110	12	174
13.	121	34	12	118	110	22	167
14.	110	34	22	121	118	12	166
15.	118	34	12	121	110	22	164
16.	110	34	12	121	118	22	156
17.	121	22	12	118	110	34	155
18.	118	22	12	121	110	34	152
19.	110	22	12	121	118	34	144
20.	34	22	12	121	118	110	68

the sum of the observations in the first (treated) group is 273. We repeat this step until all ${}^6C_3 = \binom{6}{3} = \dfrac{6.5.4}{3.2.1} = 20$ distinct rearrangements have been examined.

Five Steps to a Permutation Test

1) Analyze the problem
   a) What is the hypothesis? What are the alternatives?
   b) What distribution is the data drawn from?
   c) What losses are associated with bad decisions?
2) Choose a statistic which will distinguish the hypothesis from the alternative.
3) Compute the test statistic for the original observations.
4) Rearrange the observations
   a) Compute the test statistic for the new arrangement
   b) Compare the new value of test statistic with the value you obtained for the original observations.
   c) Repeat steps a) and b) until you are ready to make a decision.
5) Make a decision
   Reject the hypothesis and accept the alternative if the value of the test statistic for the observations as they were labelled originally is an extreme value in the permutation distribution of the statistic. Otherwise, accept the hypothesis and reject the alternative.

1.3.5. Make a Decision

The sum of the observations in the original Vitamin E treated group, 349, is equaled only once and never exceeded in the twenty distinct random re-labellings. If chance alone is operating, then such an extreme value is a rare, only-one-time-in-twenty event. I reject the null hypothesis at the five percent (1 in 20) significance level and embrace the alternative that the treatment is effective and responsible for the difference I observed.

In using this decision procedure, I risk making an error and rejecting a true hypothesis once in every twenty times. In this case, I did make just such an error. I was never able to replicate the observed life-promoting properties of Vitamin E in other repetitions of this experiment. Good statistical methods can reduce and contain the probability of making a bad decision, but they cannot eliminate the possibility.

1.4. What's in a Name?

Permutation tests are also known as randomization, rerandomization and exact tests. Historically, one may distinguish between Pitman's notion of the randomization test applicable only to the samples at hand, and Fisher's idea of a permutation test which could be applied inductively to the larger populations from which the samples are drawn, but few research workers honor this distinction today. Gabriel and Hall [1983] use the term "re-randomization" to distinguish between the initial randomization of treatment assignments at the design phase and the subsequent "rerandomizations" which occur during the permutation analysis. In this book, we shall use the three names "permutation," "randomization," and "rerandomization" interchangeably.

Most permutation tests provide "exact" significance levels. We define "exact," "significance level" and other important concepts in Section 2.3, and establish the conditions under which permutation tests are exact and unbiased. We reserve the name "exact test" for the classic Fisher's test for 2×2 tables, studying this test and other permutation tests applied to categorical data in Chapter 6.

The terms "distribution-free" and "nonparametric" often arise in connection with the permutation tests. "Distribution-free" means that the significance level of the test is independent of the form of the hypothetical infinite population from which the sample is drawn. Permutation tests are almost but not quite "distribution-free" in that only one or two assumptions about the underlying population(s) are required for their application. A preliminary rank transformation often can ensure that the tests are distribution-free. Bell and Doksum [1967] prove that all distribution-free tests of independence are permutation tests.

"Non-parametric" means that the parametric form of the underlying population distribution is not specified explicitly. It is probably safe to say that ninety-nine percent of permutation tests are nonparametric and that ninety-nine percent of common non-parametric tests are permutation tests in which the original observations have been replaced by ranks. The sign test is one notable exception.

1.4.1. Comparison with Other Tests

When the samples are very large, decisions based on parametric tests like the t-test and the F usually agree with decisions based on the corresponding permutation test. With small samples, the parametric test ordinarily is preferable IF the assumptions of the parametric test are satisfied completely. The familiar "rank" tests are simply permutation tests applied to the ranks of the observations rather than their original values, (see Sections 9.3 and 11.2).

1.4.2. Sampling from the Data at Hand

The two resampling methods—the permutation tests and the bootstrap—have much in common. Both are computer intensive, and both are limited to the data at hand.

With the permutation test, you recompute the test statistic for all possible relabelings of the combined samples. If the original samples contained the observations 1, 2, 4 and 3, 5, 6, you would consider the relabelings 1, 2, 3 and 4, 5, 6; 1, 2, 5 and 3, 4, 6 and so forth. With the bootstrap, you recompute the test statistic for each of a series of samples with replacement taken separately from each sample: thus, 1, 1, 2 and 3, 4, 4; 1, 2, 3 and 5, 5, 5 and so forth.

For some testing situations and test statistics, the bootstrap and the randomization test are asymptotically equivalent [Romano, 1989; Robinson, 1987]. But often they yield quite different results, a point we make at length in Sections 7.2 and 11.2.

When you analyze an experiment or survey with a parametric test—Student's t, for example—you compare the observed value of the test statistic with the values in a table of its theoretical distribution, for example, in a table of Student's t with eight degrees of freedom. Analyzing the same experiment with a permutation test, you compare the observed value of the test statistic with the set of what-if values you obtain by rearranging and relabeling the data.

In view of all the necessary computations—the test statistic must be recomputed for each what-if scenario—it is not surprising that the permutation test's revival in popularity parallels the increased availability of high-speed computers. Although, the permutation test was introduced by Fisher and Pitman in the 1930's, it represented initially a theoretical standard rather than a practical approach. But with each new quantum leap in computer speed, the permutation test was applied to a wider and wider variety of problems. In earlier eras—the '50's, the '60's and the '70s—the permutation test's proponents, enthusiastic at first, would grow discouraged as, inevitably, the number of computations proved too demanding for even the largest of the then-available computing machines. But with today's new and more powerful generation of desktops, it is often faster to compute a p-value for an exact permutation test than to look up an asymptotic approximation in a book of tables.

With both the bootstrap and the permutation test, all significance levels are computed on the fly. The statistician is not limited by the availability of tables, but is free to choose a test statistic exactly matched to hypothesis and alternative [Bradley, 1968].

1.5. Questions

Take the time to think about the answers to these questions even if you don't answer them explicitly.

1. In the simple example analyzed in this chapter, what would the result have been if you had used as your test statistic the difference between the sums of the first and

second samples? the difference between their means? the sum of the squares of the observations in the first sample? the sum of their ranks?

2. How was the analysis of my experiment affected by the loss of two of the cultures due to contamination? Suppose these cultures had escaped contamination and given rise to the observations 90 and 95; what would be the results of a permutation analysis applied to the new, enlarged data set consisting of the following cell counts:

Treated	121	118	110	90
Untreated	95	34	22	12

CHAPTER 2

A Simple Test

"Actually, the statistician does not carry out this very tedious process but his conclusions have no justification beyond the fact they could have been arrived at by this very elementary method."
R.A. Fisher, 1936, on permutation tests.

2.1. Properties of the Test

In this chapter, we consider the assumptions that underlie the permutation test and take a look at some of the permutation test's formal properties—its significance level, power, and robustness. This first look is relatively non-mathematical in nature. A formal derivation is provided in Chapter 14.

In the example of the missing labels in the preceding chapter, we introduced a statistical test based on the random assignment of labels to treatments. We showed this test provided a significance level of five percent, an *exact* significance level, not an approximation. The test we derived is valid under very broad assumptions. The data could have been drawn from a normal distribution or they could have come from some quite different distribution. All that is required for our permutation test comparing samples from two populations to be valid is that under the null hypothesis the distribution from which the data in the treatment group is drawn be the same as that from which the untreated sample is taken.

This freedom from reliance on numerous assumptions is a big plus. The fewer the assumptions, the fewer the limitations, and the broader the potential applications of a test. But before statisticians introduce a test into their practice, they need to know a few more things about it:

How powerful a test is it? That is, how likely is it to pick up actual differences between treated and untreated populations? Is this test as powerful or more powerful than the test we are using currently?

How robust is the new test? That is, how sensitive is it to violations in the underlying assumptions and the conditions of the experiment?

10

What if data is missing as it is in so many of the practical experiments we perform? Will missing data affect the significance level of our test?

What are the effects of extreme values or outliers? In an experiment with only five or six observations, it is obvious that a single extreme value can mislead the experimenter. In Section 9.3 of this text, you will learn techniques for diminishing the effect of extreme values.

Can we extend our results to complex experimental designs in which there are several treatments at several different levels and several simultaneous observations on each subject?

The answer to this last question, as the balance of this book will reveal to you, is yes. For example, you can easily apply permutation methods to studies in which you test a single factor at three or four levels simultaneously (see Chapter 3, Section 5). You can also apply permutation methods to experimental designs in which you control and observe the values of multiple variables (Chapters 4 and 5).

The balance of this chapter is devoted to providing a theoretical basis for all the preceding questions and answers.

2.2. Fundamental Concepts

Why do we elect to use one statistical procedure rather than another—a permutation test, say, as opposed to a table of chi-square? If you've just completed a course in statistics, you probably already know the answer. If it's been a year or so since you last looked at a statistics text, then you will find this section helpful.

In this section, you are introduced in an informal way to the fundamental concepts of variation, population and sample distributions, Type I and Type II error, significance level, power, and exact and unbiased tests. Formal definitions and derivations are provided in Chapter 14.

2.2.1. Population and Sample Distributions

The two factors that distinguish the statistical from the deterministic approach are variation and the possibility of error. The effect of this variation is that a distribution of values takes the place of a single, unique outcome.

I found Freshman Physics extremely satisfying: Boyle's Law for example, $V = KT/P$, with its tidy relationship between the volume, temperature and pressure of a perfect gas. The problem was I could never quite duplicate this law in the Freshman Physics laboratory. Maybe it was the measuring instruments, my lack of familiarity with the equipment, or simple measurement error—but I kept getting different values for the constant K.

By now, I know that variation is the norm—particularly in the clinical and biological areas. Instead of getting a fixed, reproducible V to correspond to a specific T and P, one ends up with a distribution of values instead. But I also know that, with a large enough sample, the mean and shape of this distribution are reproducible.

Figure 2.1a and 2.1b depict two such distributions. The first is a normal distribution. Examining the distribution curve, we see that the normally-distributed variable can take all possible values between $-\infty$ and $+\infty$, but most of the time it takes values that are close to its median (and mean) μ. The

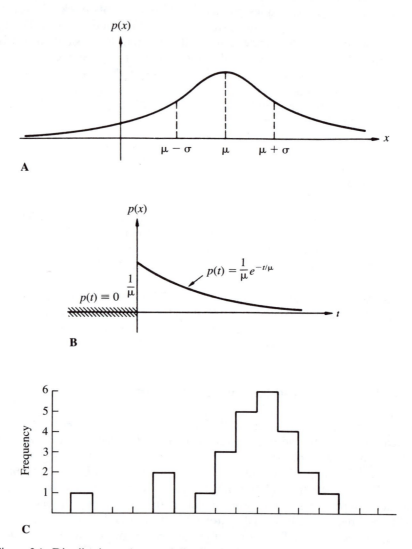

Figure 2.1. Distributions: a) normal distribution, b) exponential distribution, c) distribution of values in a sample taken from a normal distribution.

second is an exponential distribution; the exponentially-distributed variable only takes positive values; fifty percent of the time these values are less than its median μ, but on occasion they can be many times larger.

Both these distributions are limiting cases; they represent the aggregate result of an infinite number of observations; thus the distribution curves are smooth. The choppy histogram in Figure 2.1c is typical of what one sees with a small, finite sample of observations—in this case, a sample of 25 observations taken from a normal distribution with mean μ.

2.2.2. Two Types of Error

It's usually fairly easy to reason from cause to effect—that is, if you have a powerful enough computer. Get the right formula, Boyle's Law, say, plug in enough values to enough decimal places, and out pops the answer. The difficulty with reasoning in the opposite direction, from effect to cause, is that more than one set of causes can be responsible for precisely the same set of effects. We can never be completely sure which set of causes is responsible. Consider the relationship between sex (cause) and height (effect). Boys are taller than girls. Right? So that makes this new 6′2″ person in our lives ... a starter on the women's volleyball team.

In real life, in real populations, there are vast differences from person to person. Some women are tall and some women are short. In Lake Wobegon MN, all the men are good looking and all the children are brighter than average. But in most other places in the world, there is a wide range of talent and abilities. As a further example of this variation, consider that half an aspirin will usually take care of one of my headaches while other people can and do take two or three aspirins at a time and get only minimal relief.

Figure 2.2 depicts the results of an experiment in which two groups were each given a "pain-killer." The first group got buffered aspirin, the second group received a new experimental drug. Each of the participants then provided a subjective rating of the effects of the drug. The ratings ranged from "got worse," to "much improved," depicted on a scale of 0 to 4. Take a close look at Figure 2.2. Does the new drug represent an improvement over aspirin?

Those who took the new experimental drug do seem to have done better on the average than those who took aspirin. Or are the differences we observe in Figure 2.2 simply the result of chance? If it's just a chance effect and we opt in favor of the new drug, we've made an error. We also make an error if we decide there is no difference and the new drug really is better. These decisions and the effects of making them are summarized in Table 2.1.

We distinguish the two types of error because they have quite different implications. For example, Fears, Tarone, and Chu [1977] use permutation methods to assess several standard screens for carcinogenicity. Their Type I error, a false positive, consists of labeling a relatively innocuous compound

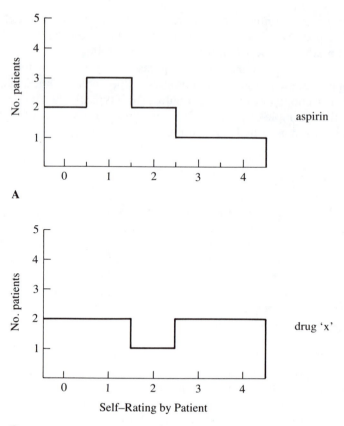

A

B

Figure 2.2. Response to treatment: self-rating by patient; a) asprin-treated group; b) drug-'x'-treated group.

Table 2.1a. Decision Making Under Uncertainty

	Our Decision	
The Facts	No Difference	Drug is better
No Difference		Type I error
Drug is Better	Type II error	

Table 2.1b. Decision Making Under Uncertainty

	Fears et al.'s Decision	
The Facts	Not a carcinogen	Compound a carcinogen
No effect		Type I error
Carcinogen	Type II error	

as carcinogenic. Such an action means economic loss for the manufacturer and the denial of the compound's benefits to the public. Neither consequence is desirable. But a false negative, a Type II error, would mean exposing a large number of people to a potentially lethal compound.

Because variation is inherent in nature, we are bound to make the occasional error when we draw inferences from experiments and surveys, particularly if, for example, chance hands us a completely unrepresentative sample. When I toss a coin in the air six times, I can get three heads and three tails, but I can also get six heads. This latter event is less probable, but it is not impossible. Does the best team always win?

We can't eliminate the risk in making decisions, but we can contain it by the correct choice of statistical procedure. For example, we can require that the probability of making a Type I error not exceed 5% (or 1% or 10%) and restrict our choice to statistical methods that ensure we do not exceed this level. If we have a choice of several statistical procedures, all of which restrict the Type I error appropriately, we can choose the method which leads to the smallest probability of making a Type II error.

2.2.3. Significance Level and Power

In selecting a statistical method, statisticians work with two closely related concepts, significance level and power. The *significance level* of a test, denoted throughout the text by the Greek letter α, is the probability of making a Type I error; that is, α is the probability of deciding erroneously on the alternative when, in fact, the hypothesis is true. The *power* of a test, denoted throughout the text by the Greek letter β, is the complement of the probability of making a Type II error; that is, β is the probability of deciding on the alternative when the alternative is the correct choice.

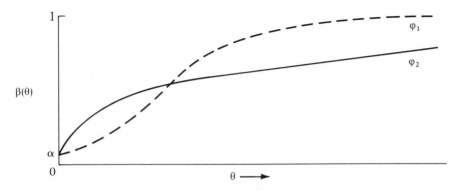

Figure 2.3. Comparing power curves. For near alternatives, with θ small, φ_2 is the more powerful test; for far alternatives, with θ large, φ_1 is more powerful. Thus neither test is uniformly most powerful.

The ideal statistical test would have a significance level α of zero and a power β of 1, or 100%. But unless we are all-knowing, this ideal can not be realized. In practice, we will fix a significance level $\alpha > 0$, where α is the largest value we feel comfortable with, and choose a statistic that maximizes or comes closest to maximizing β the power. If a test at a specific significance level α is more powerful against a specific alternative than all other tests at the same significance level, we term it *most powerful*.

As we see in Figure 2.3, the power may depend upon the alternative. In those instances when a test at a specific significance level is more powerful against all alternatives than all other tests at the same significance level, we term it *uniformly most powerful*.

The significance level and power may also depend upon how the values of the variables we observe are distributed. Does the population distribution follow a bell-shaped normal curve with the most frequent values in the center? Or is the distribution something quite different? To protect our interests, we may need to require that the Type I error be less than or equal to some predetermined value for *all* possible distributions.

Which Test Should I Use?

Figure 2.4a depicts the power curve of two tests based on samples of size 6. In this example, the ϕ_1 is uniformly more powerful than ϕ_2, hence, using ϕ_1 in preference to ϕ_2 will expose us to less risk. Figure 2.4b depicts the power curve of these same two tests but using different size samples; the power curve of ϕ_1 is still based on a sample of size 6, but that of ϕ_2 now is based on a sample of size 9. The two new power curves coincide, revealing that the two tests now have equal risks. But it would cost us 50% more observations if we were to use test 2 with its larger sample size in place of test 1.

   Moral: a more powerful test reduces the costs of experimentation while minimizing the risk.

2.2.4. Exact, Unbiased Tests

In practice, we seldom know the distribution of a variable or its variance. We usually want to test a *compound* hypothesis such as H: X has mean 0. This latter hypothesis includes several *simple* hypotheses such as H_1: X is normal with mean 0 and variance 1; H_2: X is normal with mean 0 and variance 1.2; and H_3: X has a gamma distribution with mean 0 and four degrees of freedom.

A test is said to be *exact* with respect to a compound hypothesis if the probability of making a type I error is exactly α for each and every one of the possibilities that make up the hypothesis. A test is said to be *conservative*, if the type I error never exceeds α. Obviously, an exact test is conservative though the reverse may not be true.

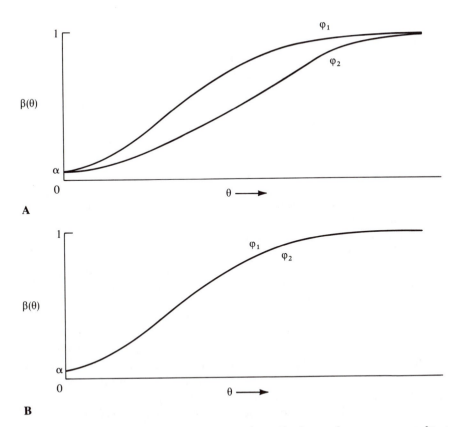

Figure 2.4. Comparing power curves. a) equal sample sizes—the power curve of test φ_1 dominates that of test φ_2. b) unequal sample sizes—the power curves of the two tests coincide.

The importance of an exact test cannot be overestimated, particularly a test that is exact regardless of the underlying distribution. If a test that is nominally at level α is actually at level χ, we may be in trouble before we start: If $\chi > \alpha$, the risk of a type I error is greater than we are willing to bear. If $\chi < \alpha$, then our test is suboptimal, and we can improve on it by enlarging its rejection region. We return to these points again in Chapter 11, on choosing a statistical method.

A test is said to be *unbiased* and of level α providing its power function β satisfies the following two conditions:

β is conservative; that is, $\beta_\theta \leq \alpha$ for every θ that satisfies the hypothesis; and

$\beta_\theta \geq \alpha$ for every θ that is an alternative to the hypothesis.

That is, a test is unbiased if using the test you are more likely to reject a false hypothesis than a true one. I find unbiasedness to be a natural and desirable principle, but not everyone shares this view; see, for example, Suissa and Shuster [1984].

Faced with some new experimental situation, our objective always is to derive a uniformly most powerful unbiased test if one exists. But, if we can't derive a uniformly most powerful test (and Figure 2.3 depicts just such a situation) then we will look for a test which is most powerful against those alternatives that are of immediate interest.

2.2.5. Exchangeable Observations

A sufficient condition for a permutation test to be exact and unbiased against shifts in the direction of higher values is the *exchangeability* of the observations in the combined sample. The observations $\{X, Y, \ldots, Z\}$ are exchangeable if the probability of any particular joint outcome, $X + Y + Z = 6$, for example, is the same regardless of the order in which the observations are considered [Lehmann 1986, p. 231]. Chapter 14, Section 1 provides a formal derivation of this fundamental result.

Independent, identically distributed observations are exchangeable. So are samples without replacement from a finite population (Polya urn models) [Koch, 1982]. So are dependent normally distributed random variables $\{X_i\}$ for which the variance of X_i is a constant independent of i and the covariance of X_i and X_j is a constant independent of i and j. An additional example of dependent but exchangeable variables is given in Section 3.4.

Sometimes a simple transformation will ensure that observations are exchangeable. For example, if we know that X comes from a population with mean μ and distribution $F(x - \mu)$ and an independent observation, Y, comes from a population with mean v and distribution $F(x - v)$, then the independent variables $X' = X - \mu$ and $Y' = Y - v$ are exchangeable.

In deciding whether your own observations are exchangeable, and whether a permutation test is applicable, the key question is the one we posed in the very first chapter, Section 1.2.2.1:

Under the null hypothesis of no differences among the various experimental or survey groups, can we exchange the labels on the observations without affecting the results?

The effect of a "no" answer to this question is discussed in Chapter 13.1 along with practical guidelines for the design and conduct of experiments and surveys to ensure the answer is "yes."

2.3. Which Test?

We are now able to make an initial comparison of the four types of statistical tests—permutation, rank, bootstrap, and parametric.

Recall from Chapter 1 that with a permutation test, we:

1. Choose a test statistic $S(X)$
2. Compute S for the original set of observations
3. Obtain the permutation distribution of S by repeatedly rearranging the observations. With two or more samples, we combine all the observations into a single large sample before we rearrange them.
4. Obtain the upper α-percentage point of the permutation distribution and accept or reject the null hypothesis according to whether S for the original observations is smaller or larger than this value.

If the observations are exchangeable than the resultant test is exact and unbiased.

As noted in this chapter's opening quotation from Fisher, although permutation tests were among the very first statistical tests to be developed, they were beyond the computing capacities of the 1930's. One alternative, which substantially reduces the amount of computation required, is the rank test. To form a rank test (e.g., Mann–Whitney or Friedman's test), we:

1. Choose a test statistic S.
2. Replace the original observations $\{X_{ij}, i = 1,\ldots,I, j = 1,\ldots,J\}$ by their ranks in the combined sample $\{R_k, k = 1\ldots IJ\}$. As an example, if the original observations are 5.2, 1, and 7, their ranks are 2, 1, and 3. Compute S for the original set of ranks.
3. Obtain the permutation distribution of S by repeatedly rearranging the ranks and recomputing the test statistic. Or, since ranks always take the same values 1, 2, and so forth, take advantage of a previously tabulated distribution.
4. Accept or reject the hypothesis in accordance with the upper α-percentage point of this permutation distribution.

In short, a rank test is simply a permutation test applied to the ranks of the observations rather than their original values. If the observations are exchangeable, then the resultant rank test is exact and unbiased. Generally, a rank test is less powerful than a permutation test, but see Section 9.3 for a discussion of the merits and drawbacks of using ranks.

The bootstrap is a relatively recent introduction (circa 1970), primarily because the bootstrap also is computation intensive. The bootstrap, like the permutation test, requires a minimum number of assumptions and derives its critical values from the data at hand.

To obtain a nonparametric bootstrap, we:

1. Choose a test statistic $S(X)$.
2. Compute S for the original set of observations.
3. Obtain the bootstrap distribution of S by repeatedly resampling from the observations. We need not combine the samples, but may resample separately from each sample. We resample with replacement.
4. Obtain the upper α-percentage point of the bootstrap distribution and accept or reject the null hypothesis according to whether S for the original observations is smaller or larger than this value.

Table 2.2. Comparison of Methods for Testing Equality of Means of Two Populations

	Distribution-free methods		
Permutation	Rank (e.g. Wilcoxon)	Nonparametric Bootstrap	Parametric (e.g. t-test)
Choose test statistic	Choose test statistic	Choose test statistic	Choose test statistic whose distribution can be derived analytically
(e.g., sum of observations in first sample)	(e.g., sum of ranks in first sample)	(e.g., difference between means of samples)	(e.g., Student's t)
Calculate statistic	Convert to ranks Calculate statistic	Calculate statistic	Calculate statistic
Are observations exchangeable?	Are observations exchangeable?	Are observations independent? With identical parameters of interest?	Are observations independent? Do they follow specified distribution?
Derive permutation distribution from combined sample	Use table of permutation distribution of ranks	Derive bootstrap distribution: resample separately from each sample	Use tabulated distribution
Compare statistic with percentiles of distribution	Compare statistic with percentiles of distribution	Compare statistic with percentiles of distribution	Compare statistic with percentiles of distribution

The bootstrap is neither exact nor conservative. Generally, but not always, a nonparametric bootstrap is less powerful than a permutation test. One exception to the rule is when we compare the variances of two populations (see Section 3.4). If the observations are independent and from distributions with identical values of the parameter of interest, then the bootstrap is asymptotically exact [Liu, 1988]. And it may be possible to bootstrap when no other statistical method is applicable, see Section 4.4.

To obtain a parametric test (e.g, a t-test or an F-test), we:

1. Choose a test statistic, S, whose distribution F_s may be computed and tabulated independent of the observations.
2. Compute S for the observations X.
3. (This step may be skipped as the distribution F_s is already known and tabulated.)

4. Compare $S(X)$ with the upper α-percentage point of F_s and accept or reject the null hypothesis according to whether $S(X)$ is smaller or larger than this value.

If S is distributed as F_s, then the parametric test is exact and, often, the most powerful test available. In order for S to have the distribution F_s, in most cases the observations need to be independent and, with small samples, identically distributed with a specific distribution, G_s. If S really has some other distribution, then the parametric test may lack power and may not be conservative. With large samples, the permutation test is usually as powerful as the most powerful parametric test [Bickel and Van Zwet, 1978]. If S is not distributed as F_s, it may be more powerful.

2.4. World Views

Parametric tests such as Student's t are based on a *sampling* model. Proponents of this model envision a hypothetical population, infinite in size, whose members take values in accordance with some fixed (if unknown) distribution function. For example, normally distributed observations would be drawn from a population whose values range from minus infinity to plus infinity in accordance with a bell-shaped or normal curve. From this population, proponents claim, we can draw a series of values of independent, identically-distributed random variables to form a random sample.

This view of the world is very natural to a trained mathematician, but does it really correspond to the practical reality which confronts the physician, the engineer, or the scientist?

Fortunately, we needn't rely on the existence of a hypothetical infinite population to form a permutation test [Welch, 1937]. The permutation tests make every bit as much sense in a context which Lehmann [1986] terms the *randomization* model in which the results are determined by the specific set of experimental subjects and by how ·these subjects are assigned to treatment.

Suppose that as a scientist you have done things or are contemplating doing things to the members of some representative subset or sample of a larger population—several cages of rats from the population of all genetically similar rats, several acres of land from the set of all similar acres, several long and twisted rods from the set of all similarly-machined rods. Or, as opposed to a sample, perhaps your particular experiment requires you to perform the same tests on every machine in your factory, or on every available fossil, or on the few surviving members of what was once—before man —a thriving species.

In these experiments, there are two sorts of variation: the variation *within* an experimental subject over which you have little or no control—blood pressure, for example, varies from hour to hour and day to day within a given individual—and the variation *between* subjects over which you have even less control. Observations on untreated subjects take on values that vary about a parameter μ_i which depends on the individual i who is being examined. Observations on treated subjects have a mean value $\mu_j + \delta$ where the treatment effect δ is confounded with the mean μ_j of the jth experimental subject. How are we to tell if the differences between observations on treated and untreated groups represent a true treatment effect or merely result from differences in the two sets of subjects?

If we assign subjects to treatment categories at *random*, so that every permutation of the labels is equally likely, the joint probability density of the observations is

$$\frac{1}{(n+m)!} \sum_{(j_1,\dots j_{m+n})} \prod_{i=1}^{m} f(x_i - \mu_{j_i}) \prod_{i=1}^{n} f(x_i - \mu_{j_{m+i}} - \delta)$$

Under the null hypothesis of no treatment effect, that is $\delta = 0$, this density can be written as

$$\frac{1}{(n+m)!} \sum_{(j_1,\dots j_{m+n})} \prod_{i=1}^{m+n} f(x_1 - \mu_{j_i})$$

By *randomizing* the assignment of subjects to treatment, we provide a statistical basis for analyzing the results. And we can reduce (but not eliminate) the probability, say, that all the individuals with naturally high blood pressure end up in the treatment group.

Because we know that blood pressure is an important factor, one that varies widely from individual to individual, we could do the experiment somewhat differently, dividing the experimental subjects into blocks so as to randomize separately within a "high" blood pressure group and a "low" blood pressure group. But we may not always know in advance which factors are important. Or, we may not be able to measure these factors until the date of the experiment itself. Fortunately, as we shall see in Sections 4.3 and 9.2, randomizing the assignment of subjects to treatment (or treatments to subject), also ensures that we are in a position to correct for significant cofactors *after* the experiment is completed.

Using a permutation test to analyze an experiment in which we have randomly assigned subjects to treatment is merely to analyze the experiment in the manner in which it was designed.

2.5. Questions

1. a) Power. Sketch the power curve $\beta(\theta)$ for one or both of the two-sample comparisons described in this chapter. (You already know two of the values for each power curve. What are they?)
   b) Using the same set of axes, sketch the power curve of a test based on a much larger sample.

c) Suppose that without looking at the data you
   i) always reject;
   ii) always accept; or
   iii) use a chance device so as to reject with probability α.
   For each of these three tests, determine the power and the significance level. Are any of these three tests exact? Unbiased?

2. a) Decisions. Suppose you have two potentially different radioactive isotopes with half-life parameters λ_1 and λ_2, respectively. You gather data on the two isotopes and, taking advantage of a uniformly-most-powerful-unbiased permutation test, you reject the null hypothesis $H: \lambda_1 = \lambda_2$ in favor of the one-sided alternative not $H: \lambda_1 > \lambda_2$. What are you or the person you are advising going to do about it? Will you need an estimate of λ_1/λ_2? What estimate will you use? (Hint: See Section 3.2 in the next chapter.)

   b) Review some of the hypotheses you tested in the past. Distinguish your actions after the test was performed from the conclusions you reached. (In other words, did you do more testing? Rush to publication? Abandon a promising line of research?) What losses were connected with your actions? Should you have used a higher/lower significance level? Should you have used a more powerful test or taken more/fewer observations? And, if you used a parametric test like Student's t or Welch's z, were all the assumptions for these tests satisfied?

CHAPTER 3

Testing Hypotheses

In this chapter, you learn how to approach and resolve a series of testing problems of increasing complexity; specifically, tests for location and scale parameters in one, two, and k samples. You learn how to derive confidence intervals for the unknown parameters. And you learn to increase the power of your tests by sampling from blocks of similar composition.

3.1. One-Sample Tests

3.1.1. Tests for a Location Parameter

One of the simplest testing problems would appear to be that of testing for the value of the location parameter of a distribution $F(\theta)$ using a series of observations $x_1, x_2, \ldots, x_n$ from that distribution. This testing problem is a simple one *if* we can assume that the underlying distribution is symmetric about the unknown parameter θ, that is, if

$$\Pr\{X \le \theta - x\} = F(\theta - x) = 1 - F(\theta + x) = \Pr\{X \ge \theta + x\}, \quad \text{for all } x.$$

The normal distribution with its familiar symmetric bell-shaped curve, and the double exponential, Cauchy, and uniform distribution are examples of symmetric distributions. The difference of two independent observations drawn from the same population also has a symmetric distribution, as you will see when we come to consider experiments involving matched pairs in Section 3.6.

Suppose we wish to test the hypothesis that $\theta \le \theta_0$ against the alternative that $\theta > \theta_0$. As in Chapter 1, we proceed in four steps:

First, we choose a test statistic that will discriminate between the hypothesis and the alternative. As one possibility, consider the sum of the deviations about θ_0. Under the hypothesis, positive and negative deviations ought to cancel and this sum should be close to zero. Under the alternative, positive terms should predominate and this sum should be large. But how large should the sum be for us to reject the hypothesis?

We saw in Chapter 2 that we can use the permutation distribution to obtain the answer; but what should we permute? The principle of sufficiency can help us here:

Suppose we had lost track of the signs (plus or minus) of the deviations. We could attach new signs at random, selecting a plus or a minus with equal probability. If we are correct in our hypothesis that the variables have a symmetric distribution about θ_0, the resulting values should have precisely the same distribution as the original observations. The absolute values of the observations are sufficient for regenerating the sample. (You'll find more on the topic of sufficiency in Sections 10.3 and 14.2 with regard to choosing a test statistic.)

Under the alternative of a location parameter larger than θ_0, randomizing the signs of the deviations should reduce the sum from what it was originally; as we consider one after another in a series of random reassignments, our original sum should be revealed as an extreme value.

Before implementing this permutation procedure, we note that the sum of just the deviations with plus signs attached is related to the sum of all the deviations by the formula:

$$\sum_{\{x_i > 0\}} x_i = (\sum x_i + \sum |x_i|)/2,$$

because the $+1$'s get added twice, once in each sum on the right hand side of the equation, whiie the -1's and $|-1|$'s cancel. Thus, we can reduce the number of calculations by summing only the positive deviations.

As an illustration, suppose that θ_0 is 0 and that the original observations are $-1, 2, 3, 1.1, 5$. Our first step is to compute the sum of the positive deviations which is 11.1.

Among the $2 \times 2 \times 2 \times 2 \times 2$ or 2^5 possible reassignments of plus and minus signs are

$$+1, \quad -2, \quad 3, \quad 1, \quad 5$$
$$+1, \quad 2, \quad 3, \quad 1, \quad 5$$

and

$$-1, \quad -2, \quad 3, \quad 1, \quad 5.$$

Our third step is to compute the sum of the positive deviations for each rearrangement. For the three rearrangements shown above, this sum would be 10, 12, and 9 respectively.

Our fourth step is to compare the original value of our test statistic with its permutation distribution. Only two of the 32 rearrangements have sums as large as the sum, 11.1, of the original observations. Is $2/32 = 1/16 = .0625$

statistically significant? Perhaps or perhaps not. It all depends on the relative losses we assign to type I and type II error and on the loss function—are small differences of practical as well as statistical significance? Certainly, a significance level of 0.0625 is suggestive. Suggestive enough that in this case we might want to look at additional data or perform additional experiments before accepting the hypothesis that 0 is the true value of θ.

3.1.2 Properties of the Test

Adopting the sampling model advanced in Section 2.4, we see the preceding permutation test is applicable even if the different observations come from different distributions—provided, that is, that these distributions are all symmetric and all have the same location parameter or median. (If these distributions are symmetric then if the mean exists, it is identical with the median.) If you are willing to specify their values through the use of a parametric model, the medians needn't be the same! (See problem 5.)

Most powerful test. Against specific normal alternatives, this permutation test provides a most powerful unbiased test of the distribution-free hypothesis $H: \theta = \theta_0$ [Lehmann, 1986, p. 239]. For large samples, its power is almost the same as Student's t-test [Albers, Bickel, and van Zwet, 1976]. We provide proofs of these and related results in Chapter 14.

Asymptotic consistency. What happens if the underlying distributions are almost but not quite symmetric? Romano [1990] shows that the permutation test for a location parameter is asymptotically exact provided the underlying distribution has finite variance. His result applies whether the permutation test is based on the mean, the median, or some statistical functional of the location parameter. If the underlying distribution is almost symmetric, the test will be almost exact even when based on as few as 10 or 12 observations. See Section 13.7 for the details of a Monte Carlo procedure to use in deciding when "almost" means "good enough."

Capsule Summary

ONE-SAMPLE TEST H: mean/median $= \theta_0$
                               K: mean/median $\neq \theta_0$
Assumptions
1) exchangeable observations
2) distributions F_i symmetric about median

Transform   Let $X_i' = X_1 - \theta_0$
Test statistic

                    Sum of nonnegative X_i'

3.1.3. Exact Significance Levels: A Digression

Many of us are used to reporting our results in terms of significance levels of 0.01, 0.05, or 0.10, and significance levels of 0.0625 or 0.03125 may seem confusing at first. These "oddball" significance levels often occur with small sample sizes. Five observations means just 32 possibilities and one extreme observation out of 32 corresponds to .03125. Things improve as sample sizes get larger. With seven observations, we can test at a significance level of .049. Is this close enough to 0.05?

Lehmann [1986] describes a method called "randomization on the boundary" for obtaining a significance level of exactly 5% (or exactly 1%, or exactly 10%). But this method isn't very practical. In the worst case, "on the boundary," you must throw a die or use some other chance device to make your decision.

What is the practical solution? We agree with Kempthorne [1975, 1977, 1979]. Forget tradition. There is nothing sacred about a p-value of 5% or 10%. Report the exact significance level, whether it is .065 or .049. Let your colleagues reach their own conclusions based on the losses they associate with each type of error.

3.2. Confidence Intervals

The method of randomization can help us find a good interval estimate of the unknown location parameter θ.

The set of confidence intervals are the duals of the corresponding tests of hypotheses:

In the first step of our permutation test for the location parameter of a single sample, we subtract θ_0 from each of the observations. We might test a whole series of hypotheses involving different values for θ_0 until we find a θ_1 such that as long as $\theta_0 \geq \theta_1$, we accept the hypothesis, but if $\theta_0 < \theta_1$ we reject it. Then an $100\,(1 - \alpha)\%$ confidence interval for θ is given by the interval $\{\theta > \theta_1\}$.

Suppose the original observations are $-1, 2, 3, 1.1$, and 5 and we want to find a confidence interval that will cover the true value of the parameter $\frac{31}{32}$nds of the time. In the first part of this chapter, we saw that $\frac{1}{16}$th of the rearrangements of the signs resulted in samples that were as extreme as these observations. Thus, we would accept the hypothesis that $\theta \leq 0$ at the $\frac{1}{16}$th and any smaller level including the $\frac{1}{32}$nd. Similarly, we would accept the hypothesis that $\theta \leq -0.5$ at the $\frac{1}{32}$nd level, or even that $\theta \leq -1 + \varepsilon$ where ε is an arbitrarily small but still positive number. But we would reject the hypothesis that $\theta \leq -1 - \varepsilon$ as after subtracting $-1 - \varepsilon$ the transformed observations are $\varepsilon, 2, 3, 1.1, 5$.

Our one-sided confidence interval is $\{-1, \infty\}$ and we have confidence that $\frac{31}{32}$nds of the time the method we've used yields an interval that includes the true value of the location parameter θ.

Our one-sided test of a hypothesis gives rise to a one-sided confidence interval. But knowing that θ is larger than -1 may not be enough. We may want to pin θ down to a more precise two-sided interval, say that θ lies between -1 and $+1$.

To accomplish this, we need to begin with a two-sided test. Our hypothesis for this test is that $\theta = \theta_0$ against the two-sided alternatives that θ is smaller or larger than θ_0. We use the same test statistic—the sum of the positive observations, that we used in the previous one-sided test. Again, we look at the distribution of our test statistic over all possible assignments of the plus and minus signs to the observations. But this time we reject the hypothesis if the value of the test statistic for the original observations is either one of the largest or one of the smallest of the possible values.

In our example, we don't have enough observations to find a two-sided confidence interval at the $\frac{31}{32}$nd level, so we'll try to find one at the $\frac{15}{16}$ths. The lower boundary of the new confidence interval is still -1. But what is the new upper boundary? If we subtract 5 from every observation, we would have the values $-6, -3, -2, -4.9, -0$; their sum is -15.9. Only the current assignment of signs to the transformed values, that is, only one out of the 32 possible assignments, yields this small a sum for the positive values. The symmetry of the permutation test requires that we set aside another $\frac{1}{32}$nd of the arrangements at the high end. Thus we would reject the hypothesis that $\theta = 5$ at the $\frac{1}{32} + \frac{1}{32}$ or $\frac{1}{16}$th level. Consequently, the interval $\{-1, 5\}$ has a $\frac{15}{16}$th chance of covering the unknown parameter value.

These results are readily extended to a confidence interval for a vector of parameters, θ, that underlies a one-sample, two-sample, or k-sample experimental design with single- or vector-valued variables. In each case, the $100(1 - \alpha)\%$ confidence interval consists of all values of the parameter vector θ for which we would accept the hypothesis at level α. Remember, one-sided tests produce one-sided intervals and two-sided tests produce two-sided confidence intervals.

In deriving a confidence interval, we look first for a *pivotal quantity* or *pivot*, $Q(X_1, \ldots, X_n, \theta)$, whose distribution is independent of the parameters of the original distribution. One example is $Q = \bar{X} - v$, where $\bar{X}$ is the sample mean, and the $\{X_i\}$ $l = 1, \ldots, n$, are independent and identically distributed as $F(x - v)$. A second example is $Q = \bar{X}/\sigma$, where the $\{X_i\}$ are independent and identically distributed as $F(x/\sigma)/\sigma$. If the $\{X_i\}$ are independent with the identical exponential distribution $1 - \exp[-\lambda t]$ (see problem 2 in Chapter 2), then $T = 2\sum t_i/\lambda$ is a pivotal quantity whose distribution does not depend on λ. We can use this distribution to find an a and b such that

$\Pr(a < T < b) = 1 - \alpha$. But then $\Pr\left\{\dfrac{1}{2b\sum t_i} < \lambda < \dfrac{1}{2a\sum t_i}\right\} = 1 - \alpha$. We use

a pivotal quantity Section 7.4 to derive a confidence interval for a regression coefficient.

For further information on deriving confidence intervals using the randomization approach see Section 14.3, as well as Lehmann [1986, pp. 246–263], Gabriel and Hsu [1983], John and Robinson [1983], Maritz [1981, p. 7,

p. 25], and Tritchler [1984]. For a discussion of the strengths and weaknesses of pivotal quantities, see Berger and Wolpert [1984].

3.2.1. Comparison with Other Tests

When a choice of statistical methods exists, the best method is the one that yields the shortest confidence interval for a given significance level. Robinson [1989] finds approximately the same coverage probabilities for three sets of confidence intervals for the slope of a simple linear regression, based, respectively, on 1) the standardized bootstrap; 2) parametric theory; and 3) a permutation procedure.

Confidence Intervals and Rejection Regions

There is a close connection between the confidence intervals and the rejection regions we've constructed. If $A(\theta')$ is a $1 - \alpha$ level acceptance region for testing the hypothesis $\theta = \theta'$, and $S(X)$ is a $1 - \alpha$ level confidence interval for θ based on the vector of observations X, then for the confidence intervals defined here, $S(X)$ consists of all the parameter values θ^* for which X belongs to $A(\theta^*)$, while $A(\theta)$ consists of all the values of the statistic x for which θ belongs to $S(x)$.

$$P_\theta\{\theta \in S(X)\} = P_\theta\{X \in A(\theta)\} \geq 1 - \alpha.$$

In Section 14.3, we show that if $A(\theta)$ is the acceptance region of an unbiased test, the correct value of the parameter is more likely to be covered by the confidence intervals we've constructed than is an incorrect value.

3.3. Two-Sample Comparisons

3.3.1. Location Parameters

We tested the equality of the location parameters of two samples in Chapter 1. Recall that we observed 121, 118, and 110 in the treatment group and 34, 12, and 22 in the control group. Our test statistic was the sum of the observations in the first group and we rejected the null hypothesis because the observed value of this statistic, 349, was as large or larger than it would have been in any of the $\binom{6}{3} = 20$ rearrangements of the data.

In Chapter 14, we show that a permutation test based on this statistic is exact and unbiased against stochastically increasing alternatives of the form $K: F_2[x] = F_1[-\delta]$, $\delta > 0$. In fact, we show that this permutation test is a uniformly most powerful unbiased test of the null hypothesis $H: F_2 = F_1$ against normally distributed shift alternatives. Against normal alternatives and for large samples, its power is equal to that of the standard t-test [Bickel and van Zwet, 1978].

The permutation test offers the advantage over the parametric t-test that it is exact even for very small samples whether or not the observations come from a normal distribution. The parametric *t*-test relies on the existence of a mythical infinite population from which all the observations are drawn (see Section 2.4). The permutation test is applicable even to finite populations such as all the machines in a given shop or all the supercomputers in the world.

3.3.2. An Example

Suppose we have two samples: The first, control sample takes values 0, 1, 2, 3, and 19. The second, treatment sample takes values 3.1, 3.5, 4, 5, and 6. Does the treatment have an effect?

The answer would be immediate if it were not for the value 19 in the first sample. The presence of this extreme value changes the mean of the first sample from 1.5 to 5. To dilute the effect of this extreme value on the results, we convert all the data to ranks, giving the smallest observation a rank of 1, the next smallest the rank of 2, and so forth. The first sample includes the ranks 1, 2, 3, 4, and 10 and the second sample includes the ranks 5, 6, 7, 8, and 9. Is the second sample drawn from a different population than the first?

Let's count. The sum of the ranks in the first sample is 15. All the rearrangements with first samples of the form 1, 2, 3, 4, k, where k is chosen from $\{5, 6, 7, 8, 9$ or $10\}$ have sums that are as small or smaller than that of our original sample. That's six rearrangements. The four rearrangements whose first sample contains 1, 2, 3, 5, and a fifth number chosen from the set $\{6, 7, 8, 9\}$ also have smaller sums. That's $6 + 4 = 10$ rearrangements so far.

Continuing in this fashion—we leave the complete enumeration as an exercise—we find that 24 of the $\binom{10}{5} = 252$ possible rearrangements have sums that are as small or smaller than that of our original sample. Two samples this different will be drawn from the same population just under ten percent of the time by chance.

Capsule Summary

TWO-SAMPLE TEST FOR LOCATION
  H: mean/medians of groups differ by d_0
  K: mean/medians of groups differ by $d > d_0$

Assumptions
  1) exchangeable observations
  2) $F_{1i}(x) = F(x) = F_{2i}(x - d)$

Transform $X'_{1i} = X_{1i} - d_0$
Test statistic
  Sum of observations in smallest sample

3.4. Comparing Variances

3.4.1. The Permutation Approach

At first glance, the permutation test for comparing the variances of two populations would appear to be an immediate extension of the test we use for
comparing the location parameters in which we use the squares of the observations rather than the observations themselves. But these squares are actually the sum of two components, one of which depends upon the unknown
variance, the other upon the unknown location parameter. In symbols, where
EX represents the mathematical expectation of a variable X:

$$EX^2 = E(X - \mu + \mu)^2 = E(X - \mu)^2 + 2\mu E(X - \mu) + \mu^2 = \sigma^2 + 0 + \mu^2.$$

A permutation test based upon the squares of the observations is appropriate
only if the location parameters of the two populations are known or are
known to be equal [Bailer, 1989].

Can't we eliminate the effects of the location parameters by working with
the deviations about each sample mean? Alas, these deviations are interdependent [Maritz, 1981]. The problem is illustrated in Figure 3.1. In the
sketch on the left, the observations in the first sample are both further from
the common center then either of the observations in the second sample, and
of the four possible rearrangements of four observations between two samples, this arrangement is the most extreme. In the sketch on the right, the
observations in the first sample have undergone a shift to the right; this shift
has altered the relative ordering of the absolute deviations about the common center, and at least one other rearrangement is more extreme.

Still, we needn't give up; if the samples are equal in size, the observations
continuous, and the two populations differ by at most a shift under the
hypothesis, we can obtain an exact permutation test with just a few preliminary calculations. First, we compute the median for each sample; e.g., in the
sample of three values—1, 6, 7—the median is 6; if there is an even number
of observations in the sample, we take as median the arithmetic average of
the two observations that bracket the median. Second, we discard the median
value from each sample; if there is an even number of observations in a
sample then we discard one of the bracketing values. Last, we replace each

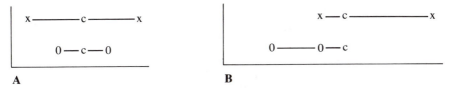

A   **B**

Figure 3.1. Comparison of two samples: a) original data, b) after first sample is shifted
to the right. c) common center, x—x first sample, 0—0 second sample.

of the remaining observations by the square of its deviation about its sample median. In the preceding example, with observations 1, 6, 7, we would be left with the squared deviates 25 and 1.

Our test statistic T is the sum of the $n - 1$ squared deviations remaining in the first sample: $T_0 = 26$ in our example. Its permutation distribution is obtained by rearranging the $2(n - 1)$ deviations remaining in the combined sample.

If under the null hypothesis the two populations differ only in their location parameters, $F_1(x) = F_2(x - \delta)$, and F is increasing over at least a semi-infinite interval, then this permutation test is exact: For the $n - 1$ deviations remaining in the first sample are mutually exchangeable as are the $n - 1$

Capsule Summary

TWO-SAMPLE TEST FOR VARIANCE
  H: variances of populations are equal
  K: $\sigma_2^2 > \sigma_1^2$

Assumptions
  1) independent observations
  2) continuous observations
  3) $F_{1i}(x) = F_{2i}(x - d)$

Transform $X'_{ij} = (X_{ij} - Mdn_i)^2$
  discard redundant deviate from each sample

Test statistic
  Sum of X'_{ij} in smallest sample

---

deviations remaining in the second sample. The shift relation between the two populations ensures that the two sets of deviations are jointly exchangeable. Exactness follows.

Although there are several dozen alternate solutions to the problem of comparing the variances of two populations (see, for example, the list in Conover, Johnson and Johnson [1981]), in a recent series of computer simulations, my friend Michael Chernick and I found that none are close to exact for samples of under sixteen in size. The permutation test for comparing variances is exact, powerful, and distribution free.

3.4.2. The Bootstrap Approach

In order to use permutation methods to compare the variances of two populations, we have to sacrifice two of the observations. The resultant test is exact and distribution free, but it is not most powerful. A more powerful test is provided by the bootstrap confidence interval for the variance ratio. To

Table 3.1A. Significance levels for Variance Comparisons for BC_a method, Efron and Tibshirani [X: 1986].* For various underlying distributions by sample size. 500 simulations.

	6, 6	8, 8	8, 12	12, 8	12, 12	15, 15
Ideal	50	50	50	50	50	50
normal (0, 1)	44	52	53	56	45	49
double (0, 1)	53	51	63	70	55	54
gamma (4. 1)	48	55	60	65	52	52
exponential	54	58	56	70	46	63

* X preceding a date, as in Efron, X:1986, refers to a supplemental bibliography at the end of the text which includes material not directly related to permutation methods

Table 3.1B. Power as a Function of the Ratio of the Variances. For various distributions and two samples each of size 8. Rejections in 500 Monte Carlo simulations.

	permutation test					bootstrap*				
$\phi = \sigma_2/\sigma_1$	1.	1.5	2.	3.	4.	1.	1.5	2.	3.	4.
Ideal	50				500	50			444	500
normal	52	185	312	438	483	52	190	329	379*	482
double	55	153	215	355	439	53	151*	250*	426	433
gamma	44	158	255	411	462	49	165	288	344*	464
exponential	51	132	224	323	389	54	150*	233*		408

* bootstrap intervals shortened so actual significance level is 10%.

derive this test, we resample repeatedly without replacement, drawing independently from the two original samples, until we have two new samples the same size as the originals. Each time we resample, we compute the variances of the two new independent subsamples and calculate their ratio. The resultant bootstrap confidence interval is asymptotically exact [Efron, 1981] and can be made close to exact with samples of as few as eight observations: See Table 3.1A. As Table 3.1B shows, this bootstrap is more powerful than the permutation test we described in the previous section. One caveat also revealed in the table: this bootstrap is still only "almost" exact.

3.5. k-Sample Comparisons

3.5.1. F-Ratio

Just as Student's t is the classic parametric statistic for testing the hypothesis that the means of two normal distributions are the same, so the F-ratio of the between-group variance to the within-group variance is the classic parametric statistic for testing the hypothesis that the means of k normal distributions are the same [Welch, 1937; Pitman, 1937].

Explicitly, let X_{ij} ($j = 1,\ldots,n_i$; $i = 1,\ldots,s$) be independently distributed as $F(x - \mu_i)$, and thus exchangeable, and consider the hypothesis $H\colon \mu_1 = \cdots = \mu_s$, and the alternative not $H\colon \mu_i \neq \mu_j$ for some pair (i, j). Welch [1937] proposes as test statistic

$$W = \frac{\sum n_i(X_i. - X..)^2/(s - 1)}{\sum\sum(X_{ij} - X_i.)^2/(n - s)} \tag{3.5.1}$$

It is easy to see that W is invariant under transformations of scale or origin. Lehmann [1986, p. 375] shows that against normal alternatives, and among all similarly invariant tests, the parametric test based on W is a uniformly most powerful procedure.

If the X_{ij} are normally distributed with a common variance, then under the hypothesis, W has the F-distribution with $s - 1$, $n - s$ degrees of freedom. But we may not know or not be willing to assume that these observations do come from a normal distribution. Since the observations are independent and identically distributed, they are exchangeable and, whether or not they are normally distributed, we can still obtain the permutation distribution of W. We examine all possible reassignments of the observations to the various treatment groups subject to the restriction that the number of observations in each of the k groups remains unchanged. Our analysis is exact if the experimental units were randomly assigned to treatment to begin with.

In a sidebar, we've provided an outline of a computer program that uses a Monte Carlo to estimate the significance level (see Section 13.2). This program is applicable to any of the experimental designs we consider in this chapter and the next. Our one programing trick is to pack all the observations into a single linear vector $X = (X_{11},\ldots,X_{1n_1},X_{1n_1+1},\ldots,X_{1n_1+n_2},\ldots)$ and then to permute the observations within the vector. If we have k samples, we only need to select $k - 1$ of them when we rearrange the data. The kth sample is left over automatically.

We need to write a subprogram to compute the test statistic but there's less work involved than the formula for W would suggest. As is the case with the permutation equivalent of the t-statistic, we can simplify the calculation of the test statistic by eliminating terms that are invariant under permutation of the subscripts. For example, the *within-group* sum of squares in the denominator of W may be written as two sums $\sum\sum(X_{ij} - X..)^2$ and $\sum n_i(X_i. - X..)^2$. The first of these sums is invariant under permutation of the subscripts. The second, the *between-groups* sum of squares, already occurs in the numerator. Our test statistic reduces to the between-groups sum of squares

---

Sidebar

Program for estimating permutation significance levels; for tips on optimization, see Chapter 12.

    Monte, the number of Monte Carlo simulations; try 400
    S_0, the value of the test statistic for the unpermuted observations
    S, the value of the test statistic for the rearranged observations
    $X[\ ]$, a one-dimensional vector that contain the observations
    $n[\ ]$, a vector that contains the sample sizes
    N, the total number of observations

Main program
    Get data
        put all the observations into a single linear vector
    Compute the test statistic S_0
    Repeat Monte times:
        Rearrange the observations
        Recompute the test statistic S
        Compare S with S_0
    Print out the proportion of times S was equal to or larger than S_0

Rearrange
    Set s to the size of the combined sample
    Start: Choose a random integer k from 0 to $s - 1$
        Swap $X[k]$ and $X[s - 1]$:
          temp   = $X[k]$;
          $X[k]$ = $X[s - 1]$;
          $X[s - 1]$ = temp.
        Decrement s and repeat from start
    Stop after you've selected all but one of the samples.

Get data
    This user-written procedure gets all the data and packs it into a single long
        linear vector X.

Compute stat
    This user-written procedure computes the test statistic.

$$\sum n_i(X_{i.} - X_{..})^2$$

with a corresponding reduction in the number of calculations.

The size and power of this test are robust in the face of violations of the normality assumption providing that the $\{X_{ij}; j = 1, \ldots, n_i\}$ are samples from distributions $F(x - \mu_i)$ where F is an arbitrary distribution with finite variance [Robinson, 1973, 1983]. However, the parametric version of the test is almost as robust. The real value of the permutation approach comes when we realize that we are not restricted to a permutation version of an existing statistic but are free to choose a test statistic optimal for the problem at hand.

3.5.2. Pitman Correlation

The F-ratio test and its permutation version offer protection against any and all deviations from the null hypothesis of equality among treatment means. As a result, they may offer less protection against some specific alternative than some other test function(s). When we have a specific alternative in mind, as is so often the case in biomedical research; for example, when we are testing for an ordered dose response, the F-ratio may not be the statistic of choice.

Frank, Trzos, and Good [1977] studied the increase in chromosome abnormalities and micronucleii as the dose of various known mutagens was increased. Their object was to develop an inexpensive but sensitive biochemical test for mutagenicity that would be able to detect even marginal effects. Thus they were more than willing to trade the global protection offered by the F-test for a statistical test that would be sensitive to ordered alternatives.

Fortunately, a most powerful unbiased test (and one that is also most powerful among tests that are invariant to changes in scale) has been known since the late 1930's. Pitman [1937] proposes a test for linear correlation using as test statistic

$$S = \sum f[i] n_i X_i$$

where $f[i]$ is any monotone increasing function. The simplest choice is $f[i] = i$.

The permutation distributions of S_1 with $f[i] = ai + b$ and S_2 with $f[i] = i$ are equivalent in the sense that if S_{10}, S_{20} are the values of these test statistics corresponding to the same set of observations $\{x_i\}$, then $\Pr(S_1 > S_{10}) = \Pr(S_2 > S_{20})$.

Let us apply the Pitman approach to the data collected by Frank et al. shown in Table 3.2. As the anticipated effect is proportional to the logarithm of the dose, we take

$f[\text{dose}] = \log[\text{dose} + 1]$. (Adding a 1 to the dose keeps this function from blowing up at a dose of zero.) There are four dose groups; the original data for breaks may be written in the form

Table 3.2. Micronucleii in polychromatophilic erythrocytes and chromosome alterations in the bone marrow of mice treated with CY.

Dose (mg/kg)	Number of animals	Micronucleii per 200 cells	Breaks per 25 cells
0	4	0 0 0 0	0 1 1 2
5	5	1 1 1 4 5	0 1 2 3 5
20	4	0 0 0 4	3 5 7 7
80	5	2 3 5 11 20	6 7 8 9 9

0 1 1 2   0 1 2 3 5   3 5 7 7   6 7 8 9 9

As $\log[0 + 1] = 0$, the value of the Pitman statistic for the original data is

$0 + 11 * \log[6] + 22 * \log[21] + 39 * \log[81] = 112.1$. The only larger values are associated with the small handful of rearrangements of the form

0 0 1 2	1 1 2 3 5	3 5 7 7	6 7 8 9 9
0 0 1 1	1 2 2 3 5	3 5 7 7	6 7 8 9 9
0 0 1 1	1 2 2 3 3	5 5 7 7	6 7 8 9 9
0 0 1 2	1 1 2 3 3	5 5 7 7	6 7 8 9 9
0 1 1 2	0 1 2 3 3	5 5 7 7	6 7 8 9 9
0 1 1 2	0 1 2 3 5	3 5 6 7	7 7 8 9 9
0 0 1 2	1 1 2 3 5	3 5 6 7	7 7 8 9 9
0 0 1 1	1 2 2 3 5	3 5 6 7	7 7 8 9 9
0 0 1 1	1 2 2 3 3	5 5 6 7	7 7 8 9 9
0 0 1 2	1 1 2 3 3	5 5 6 7	7 7 8 9 9
0 1 1 2	0 1 2 3 3	5 5 6 7	7 7 8 9 9

A statistically significant ordered dose response ($\alpha < 0.001$) has been detected. The micronucleii also exhibit a statistically significantly dose response when we calculate the permutation distribution of $S = \sum \log[\text{dose}_i + 1]n_i X_i.$. To make the calculations, we took advantage of the computer program we developed in Section 3.6.1; the only change was in the subroutine used to compute the test statistic.

A word of caution: If we use some function of the dose other than $f[\text{dose}] = \log[\text{dose} + 1]$, we might not observe a statistically significant result. Our choice of a test statistic must always make biological as well as statistical sense; see question 3 in Section 3.9.

3.5.3. Effect of Ties

Ties can complicate the determination of the significance level. Because of ties, each of the rearrangements noted in the preceding example might actually have resulted from several distinct reassignments of subjects to treatment groups and must be weighted accordingly. To illustrate this point, suppose we put tags on the 1's in the original sample

0 1* 1# 2   0 1 2 3 5   3 5 7 7   6 7 8 9 9

The rearrangement

0 0 1 2   1 1 2 3 5   3 5 7 7   6 7 8 9 9

corresponds to the three reassignments

0 0 1	2	1* 1# 2 3 5	3 5 7 7	6 7 8 9 9	
0 0 1*	2	1 1# 2 3 5	3 5 7 7	6 7 8 9 9	
0 0 1#	2	1 1* 2 3 5	3 5 7 7	6 7 8 9	

The 18 observations are divided into four dose groups containing 4, 5, 4, and 5 observations respectively so that there are $\binom{18}{4\ 5\ 4\ 5}$ possible reassignments of observations to dose groups. Each reassignment has probability $\dfrac{1}{\binom{18}{4\ 5\ 4\ 5}}$ of occurring so the probability of the rearrangement

$$0\ 0\ 1\ 2 \qquad 1\ 1\ 2\ 3\ 5 \qquad 3\ 5\ 7\ 7 \qquad 6\ 7\ 8\ 9\ 9$$

is

$$\frac{3}{\binom{18}{4\ 5\ 4\ 5}}.$$

To determine the significance level when there are ties, weight each distinct rearrangement by its probability of occurrence. This weighting is done automatically if you use Monte Carlo sampling methods as is done in the computer program we provide in section 3.6.1.

Capsule Summary

K-SAMPLE TEST
   H: all distributions and, in particular,
      all population means the same
   K1: at least one pair of means differ
   K2: the population means are ordered

Assumptions
   1) exchangeable observations
   2) $F_{ij}(x) = F(x - \mu_i)$

Transform   None
Test statistic
   K1: $\sum n_i(X_{i.} - X_{..})^2$.
   K2: $\sum f[i]n_i X_{i.}$.

3.5.4. Linear Estimation

Pitman correlation may be generalized by replacing the fixed function $f[i]$ by an estimate $\hat{\phi}$ derived by a linear estimation procedure such as least squares polynomial regression, kernel estimation, local regression, and smoothing splines [Raz, 1990].

Suppose the jth treatment group is defined by x_j, a vector-valued design variable (x_j might include settings for temperature, humidity, and phosphorous concentration). Suppose also that we may represent the ith observation in the jth group by a regression model of the form

$$Y_{ji} = \mu(x_j) + e_{ji}, \qquad j = 1, \ldots, n$$

where e is an error variable with mean 0, and $\mu(x)$ is a smooth regression function (that is, for any x and ε sufficiently small, $\mu(x + \varepsilon)$ may be closely approximated by the first-order Taylor expansion $\mu(x) + b\varepsilon$).

The null hypothesis is that $\mu(x) = \mu$, a constant that does not depend on the design variable x. As always, we assume that the errors e_{ji} are exchangeable so that all $n!$ assignments of the labels to the observations that preserve the sample sizes $\{n_j\}$ are equally likely.

Raz's test statistic is $Q = \sum (\hat{\mu}(x_j))^2$ where $\hat{\mu}$ is an estimate of μ derived by a linear estimation procedure such as least squares polynomial regression, kernel estimation, local regression, and smoothing splines.

This test may be performed using the permutation distribution of Q or, for large samples, a gamma-distribution approximation. See also Section 7.3.

3.5.5. A Unifying Theory

The permutation tests for Pitman correlation and the two-sample comparison of means are really special cases of a more general class of tests that take the form of a dot product of two vectors [Wald and Wolfowitz, 1947; De Cani, 1979]. Let $W = \{W_1, \ldots, W_N\}$ and $Z = \{Z_1, \ldots, Z_N\}$ be fixed sets of numbers and let $z = \{z_1, \ldots, z_N\}$ be a random permutation of the elements of Z. Then we may use the dot product of the vectors z and W, $T = \sum z_i w_i$, to test the hypothesis that the labelling is irrelevant. In the two-sample comparison, W is a vector of m 1's followed by n 0's. In Pitman correlation, $W = \{f[1], \ldots, f[N]\}$ where f is a monotone function.

3.6. Blocking

Although the significance level of a permutation test may be "distribution-free," its power strongly depends on the underlying distribution.

Figure 3.2 depicts the effect of a change in the variance of the underlying population on the power of the permutation test for the difference in two means. As the variance increases, the power decreases. *To get the most from your experiments, reduce the variance.*

One way to reduce the variance is to subdivide the population under study into more homogeneous subpopulations and to take separate samples from each. Suppose you were designing a survey on the effect of income level on the respondents' attitudes toward compulsory pregnancy. Obviously, the

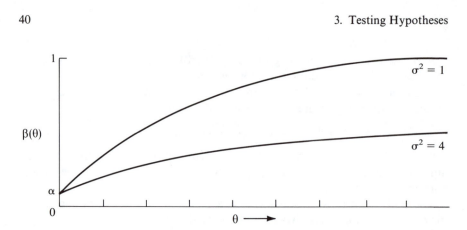

Figure 3.2. Effect of the population variance on the power of a test of two means. $\theta = \theta_1 - \theta_2$.

views of men and women differ markedly on this controversial topic. It would not be prudent to rely on randomization to even out the sex ratios in the various income groups.

The recommended solution is to block the experiment, to interview, and to report on, men and women separately. You would probably want to do the same type of blocking in a medical study. Similarly, in an agricultural study, you would want to distinguish among clay soils, sandy, and sandy-loam.

In short, whenever a population can be subdivided into distinguishable subpopulations, you can reduce the variance of your observations and increase the power of your statistical tests by blocking or stratifying your sample.

Suppose we have agreed to divide our sample into two blocks—one for men, one for women. If this is an experiment, rather than a survey, we would then assign subjects to treatments separately within each block.

In a study that involves two treatments and ten experimental subjects, four men and six women, we would first assign the men to treatment and then the women. We could assign the men in any of $\binom{4}{2} = 6$ ways and the women in any of $\binom{6}{3} = 20$ ways. That is, there are $6 \times 20 = 120$ possible random assignments in all.

When we come to analyze the results of our experiment, we use the permutation approach to ensure we analyze in the way the experiment was designed. Our test statistic is a natural extension of that used for the two-sample comparison [Lehmann, 1986], pp. 233–4:

$$S = \sum_{b=1}^{B} \sum_{j=m_b+1}^{(n_b+m_b)} x_{bj} \tag{3.6.1}$$

where B is the number of blocks, two in the present example, and the inner sum extends over the n_b treated observations x_{bj} within each block.

We compute the test statistic for the original data. Then, we rearrange the observations at random within each block, subject to the restriction that the number of observations within each treatment category—the pair $\{n_b, m_b\}$—remain constant.

We compute S for each of the 120 possible rearrangements. If the value of S for the original data is among the 120α largest values, then we reject the null hypothesis; otherwise we accept it.

3.6.1. Extending the Range of Applications

The resulting permutation test is exact and most powerful against normal alternatives even if the observations on men and women have different distributions [Lehmann, 1986]. As we saw in Section 2.3, all that is required is that the subsets of errors be exchangeable.

The design need not be balanced. The test statistic S (equation 3.6.1) is a sum of sums. Unequal sample sizes resulting from missing data or an inability to complete one or more portions of the experiment will affect the analysis only in the relative weights assigned to each subgrouping.

Warning: This remark applies only if the data is missing at random. If treatment-related withdrawals are a problem in one of your studies, see Entsuah [1990] for the details of a resampling procedure.

Blocking is applicable to any number of subgroups; in the extreme case, that in which every pair of observations forms a distinct subgroup, we have the case of matched pairs.

3.7. Matched Pairs

In a matched pairs experiment, we take blocking to its logical conclusion. Each subject in the treatment group is matched as closely as possible by a subject in the control group. For example, if a 45-year old black male hypertensive is given a blood-pressure lowering pill, then we give a second similarly-built 45-year old black male hypertensive a placebo. One member of each pair is then assigned at random to the treatment group, and the other member is assigned to the controls.

Assuming we have been successful in our matching, we will end up with a series of independent pairs of observations (X_i, Y_i) where the members of each pair have been drawn from the distributions $F_i(x - v)$ and $F_i(x - v - \delta)$ respectively. Regardless of the form of this unknown distribution, the differences $Z_i = Y_i - X_i$ will be symmetrically distributed about the unknown parameter δ:

$$\Pr(Z \le z + \delta) = \Pr\{Y - X \le z + \delta\}$$
$$= \Pr\{(Y - v) - (X - v) \le z + \delta\}$$
$$= \int \Pr\{Y - v = z + \delta + s\} \Pr\{X - v = s\}\, ds$$

$$= \int F(z + s)f(s)\,ds$$

$$= \int \Pr\{X - v = z + s\}\Pr\{Y - v - \delta = s\}\,ds$$

$$= \Pr\{(X - v) - (Y - v - \delta) \le z\}$$

$$= \Pr\{X - Y \le z - \delta\}$$

$$= \Pr\{Y - X \ge -z + \delta\}$$

$$= \Pr(Z \ge -z + \delta)$$

This is precisely the case we considered at the beginning of this chapter and the same readily computed permutation test is applicable.

This permutation test has the same properties of exactness, lack of bias, and sensitivity under the same conditions as the one-sample test with the following exception: If the observation on one member of a pair is missing, then we must discard the remaining observation.

For an almost most powerful test when one member of the pair is censored, see Section 9.4. For an application of a permutation test to the case where an experimental subject serves as her own control, see Shen and Quade [1986].

Capsule Summary

MATCHED-PARIS
  H: distributions and, in particular, means/medians of the members of each pair
    are the same
  K: means/medians of the members of each pair differ by $d > 0$

Assumptions
  1) independent observations
  2) $F_{1i}(x) = F_{2i}(x - d)$

Transform $z_i = x_{1i} - x_{2i}$
Test statistic   Sum of positive z_i

3.8. Questions

1. Show that the following statistics lead to equivalent permutation tests for the equality of two location parameters:
   a) $\sum X_{2i}$ (our original choice)
   b) $\sum X_{2i}/n_2 - \sum X_{1i}/n_1$ (the difference of the sample means)

   c) $\dfrac{(\sum X_{2i}/n_2 - \sum X_{1i}/n_1)}{\sqrt{(\sum(X_{2i} - X_{2\cdot})^2 + \sum(X_{1i} - X_{1\cdot})^2)/(m + n - 2)}}$ (the t-statistic).

Hint: The sums $(\sum X_{2i} + \sum X_{1i})$, $(\sum X_{2i}^2 + \sum X_{2i}^2)$ and the sample sizes n_1, n_2 are invariant under permutations.

2. In the example of Section 3.3.2, list all rearrangements in which the sum of the ranks in the first sample is less than or equal to the original sum.

3. Use both the F-ratio and Pitman correlation to analyze the data for micronucleii in Table 3.2. Explain the difference in results.

4. The following vaginal virus titres were observed in mice by H.E. Renis of the Upjohn Company 144 hours after inoculation with Herpes virus type II (see Good [1979] for complete details):

Saline controls	10000,	3000,	2600,	2400,	1500.
Treated with antibiotic	9000,	1700,	1100,	360.,	1.

Is this a one-sample, two-sample, k-sample, or matched pairs study? Does treatment have an effect?

Most authorities would suggest using a logarithmic transformation before analyzing this data. Repeat your analysis after taking the logarithm of each of the observations. Is there any difference? Compare your results and interpretations with those of Good [1979].

5. Using the logarithm of the viral titre, determine an approximate 90% confidence interval for the treatment effect. (Hint: Keep subtracting a constant from the logarithms of the observations on saline controls until you can no longer detect a treatment difference.)

6. Suppose you make a series of I independent *pairs* of observations $\{x_i, y_i; i = 1\ldots I\}$. y_i might be tensile strength and x_i the percentage of some trace metal. You know from your previous work that each of the y_i has a symmetric distribution.
   a) How would you test the hypothesis that for all i, the median of y_i is x_i? (Hint: See 3.1.2.)
   b) Do you need to assume that the distributions of the $\{y_i\}$ all have the same shape, i.e., that they are all normal or all double exponential? Are the $\{y_i\}$ exchangeable? Are the $\{z_i = y_i - x_i\}$? (We return to these questions in Chapter 7.)

CHAPTER 4

Experimental Designs

4.1. Introduction

In this chapter, we explore the use of permutation methods for analyzing the results of complex experimental designs that may involve multiple control variables, covariates, and restricted randomization.

4.2. Balanced Designs

The analysis of randomized blocks we studied in Chapter 3 can be generalized to very complex experimental designs with multiple control variables and confounded effects. In this section, we consider the evaluation of main effects and interactions in the two- and three-way univariate analysis of variance and in the Latin Square. Only *balanced* designs with the sample sizes equal in all subcategories are considered here. Unbalanced designs are considered in Section 4.4.

What distinguishes the complex experimental design from the simple one-sample, two-sample, and k-sample experiments we have considered so far is the presence of *multiple* control factors.

For example, we may want to assess the simultaneous effects on crop yield of hours of sunlight and rainfall. We determine to observe the crop yield X_{ijm} for I different levels of sunlight, $i = 1, \ldots, I$, and J different levels of rainfall, $j = 1, \ldots, J$, and to make M observations at each factor combination, $m = 1, \ldots, M$. We adopt as our model relating the dependent variable, crop-yield (the effect) to the independent variables of sunlight and rainfall (the causes)

$$X_{ijm} = \mu + s_i + r_j + (sr)_{ij} + \varepsilon_{ijm}.$$

In this model, terms with a single subscript like s_i, the effect of sunlight, are called *main effects*. Terms with multiple subscripts like sr_{ij}, the residual and nonadditive effect of sunlight and rainfall, are called *interactions*. The $\{\varepsilon_{ijm}\}$ represent that portion of crop yield that can not be explained by the independent variables alone; these are variously termed the residuals, the errors, or the model errors. To ensure the residuals are exchangeable so that permutation methods can be applied, the experimental units must be assigned at random to treatment (see Section 4.2.5).

If we wanted to assess the simultaneous effect on crop yield of three factors simultaneously—sunlight, rainfall, and fertilizer, say, we would observe the crop yield X_{ijkm} for I different levels of sunlight, $i = 1, \ldots, I$, J different levels of rainfall, $j = 1, \ldots, J$, and K different levels of fertilizer, $k = 1, \ldots, K$ and make M observations at each factor combination, $m = 1, \ldots, M$. Our model would then be

$$X_{ijkm} = \mu + s_i + r_j + f_k + (sr)_{ij} + (s)_{ik} + (r)_{jk} + (sr)_{ijk} + \varepsilon_{ijkm}.$$

In this model we have three main effects, s_i, r_j, and f_k, three two-way interactions, $(sr)_{ij}$, $(s)_{ik}$, $(r)_{jk}$, a single three-way interaction, $(sr)_{ijk}$, and the error term ε_{ijkm}.

Including the additive constant μ in the model allows us to define all main effects and interactions so they sum to zero,

$$\sum s_i = 0,$$

$$\sum_i (sr)_{ij} = 0 \quad \text{for} \quad j = 1, \ldots, J,$$

and so forth. That is, under the null hypothesis of no effect of sunlight on crop yield, each of the main effects $s_1 = \cdots = s_I = 0$. Under the alternative, the different terms s_i represent deviations from a zero average, with the interaction term $(sr)_{ij}$ representing the deviation from the sum $s_i + r_j$.

Clearly, when we have multiple factors, we must also have multiple test statistics. In the preceding example, we require three separate tests and test statistics for the three main effects s_i, r_j, and f_k, plus four other statistical tests for the three two-way and the one three-way interactions. Will we be able to find statistics that measure a single intended effect without confounding it with a second unrelated effect? Will the several test statistics be independent of one another?

In the permutation analysis of an experimental design as in the parametric analysis of variance, the answer is yes to both questions only if the design is balanced, that is, if there are equal numbers of observations in each subcategory, and if the test statistics are independent of one another.

In a balanced design, the permutation test has a three-fold advantage over the parametric ANOVA: it is exact; it is not restricted by an assumption of normality (although, it does require that the experimental errors be exchangeable; see Section 2.2); yet it is as powerful or more powerful than parametric approach; see Scheffe 1959; Collier and Baker, 1966; and Bradbury, 1987.

In an unbalanced design, main effects will be *confounded* with interactions so that the two cannot be tested separately, a topic we return to in Section 4.5.

4.2.1. Main Effects

In a k-way analysis with equal sample sizes M in each category, we can assess the main effects using essentially the same statistics we would use for randomized blocks. Take sunlight in the preceding example. If we have only two levels of sunlight, then, referring to equation 3.6.1, our test statistic for the effect of sunlight is

$$S = \sum_{j=1}^{J} \sum_{k=1}^{K} \sum_{m=1}^{M} X_{1jkm} \tag{4.1}$$

If we have more than two levels of sunlight, our test statistic is

$$F2 = \sum_{i=1}^{I} \sum_{j=1}^{J} \sum_{k=1}^{K} (X_{ijk\cdot} - X_{\cdot jk\cdot})^2 \tag{4.2}$$

or

$$F1 = \sum_{i=1}^{I} \sum_{j=1}^{J} \sum_{k=1}^{K} |X_{ijk\cdot} - X_{\cdot jk}| \tag{4.3}$$

The dot . used as a subscript indicates that we have summed over the corresponding subscript and then taken an average by dividing by the number of terms in that sum; thus

$$X_{ijk\cdot} = \sum_{m=1}^{M} X_{ijkm}/M.$$

The statistics F2 and F1 offer protection against a broad variety of shift alternatives including

$$K_1: s_1 = s_2 > s_3 = \cdots$$

$$K_2: s_1 > s_2 > s_3 = \cdots$$

$$K_3: s_1 < s_2 > s_3 = \cdots$$

As a result, they may not provide a most powerful test for any single one of these alternatives. If we believe the effect to be monotone increasing, then, in line with the thinking detailed in Section 3.5, we would use the Pitman correlation statistic

$$R = \sum_{i=1}^{I} \sum_{j=1}^{J} \sum_{k=1}^{K} f[i](X_{ijk\cdot} - X_{\cdot jk\cdot}) \tag{4.4}$$

To obtain the permutation distributions of the test statistics S, F2, F1, and R, we permute the observations independently in each of the JK blocks determined by a specific combination of rainfall and fertilizer. Exchanging observations *within* a category corresponding to a specific level of sunlight leaves the statistics S, F2, F1, and R unchanged. We can concentrate on exchanges *between* categories, and the total number of rearrangements is

$$\binom{M}{M \ldots M}^{JK}.$$

We compute the test statistic (S, F1, or R) for each rearrangement, rejecting the hypothesis that sunlight has no effect on crop yield only if the value of S (or F1 or R) that we obtain using the original arrangement of the observations lies among the α most extreme of these values.

Of the two F-statistics, F1 is to be preferred to F2. F1 is as powerful or more powerful for detecting location shifts and more powerful for detecting concentration changes [Mielke and Berry, 1983].

A third alternative to F1 and F2 is

$$F_3 = \sum \frac{n_j(n_j - 1)(X_{j.} - X_{..})^2}{\sum_k (X_{jk} - X_{j.})^2} \tag{4.5}$$

[James, 1951] which Hall [1989] recommends for use with the bootstrap when we can not be certain that the observations in the various categories all have the same variance. In simulation studies with permutation tests and variances that differed by an order of magnitude, I found F3 was inferior to F1.

A final alternative to the statistics S, F1, and F2 is the standard F-ratio statistic

$$F = \frac{\sum_{i=1}^{I} M_i(X_{i..} - X_{...})^2}{(I - 1)\hat{\sigma}^2} \tag{4.6}$$

where $\hat{\sigma}^2$ is our estimate of the variance of the errors ε_{ijk}. But if we use F, we are forced to consider exchanges between as well as within blocks, thus negating the advantages of blocking as described in Section 3.5.

4.2.2. An Example

In this section, we apply the permutation method to determine the main effects of sunlight and fertilizer on crop yield using the data from the two-factor experiment depicted in Table 4.1a. As there are only two levels of sunlight in this experiment, we use S (equation 4.1) to test for the main effect. For the original observations, $S = 23 + 55 + 75 = 153$. One possible rearrangement is shown in Table 4.1b in which we have interchanged the two observations marked with an asterisk, the 5 and 6. The new value of S is 154.

As can be seen by a continuing series of straightforward hand calculations, the test statistic, S, for the main effect of sunlight is as small or smaller than it is for the original observations in only 8 out of the $\binom{6}{3}^3 = 8000$ possible rearrangements. For example, it is smaller when we swap the 9 of the Hi-Lo group for the 10 of the Lo-Lo group (the two observations marked with the pound sign). As a result, we conclude that the effect of sunlight is statistically significant.

The computations for the main effect of fertilizer are more complicated —we must examine $\binom{9}{3\ 3\ 3}^2$ rearrangements, and compute the statistic F1

Table 4.1a. Effect of Sunlight and Fertilizer
on Crop Yield

		Fertilizer		
S		LO	MED	HIGH
u	LO	5	15	21
n		10	22	29
l		8	18	25
i				
g	HI	6	25	55
h		9	32	60
t		12	40	48

Table 4.1b. Effect of Sunlight and
Fertilizer. Data Rearranged

	LO	MED	HIGH
LO	6*	15	21
	10 #	22	29
	8	18	25
HI	5*	25	55
	9 #	32	60
	12	40	48

for each. We use F1 rather than R because of the possibility that too much fertilizer—the "High" level, might actually suppress growth. Only a computer can do this many calculations quickly and correctly, so we adapted our program from Section 3.4 to make them (see Sidebar). The estimated significance level is .001 and we conclude that this main effect, too, is statistically significant.

In this last example, each category held the same number of experimental subjects. If the numbers of observations were unequal, our main effect would have been confounded with one or more of the interactions (see Section 4.5). In contrast to the simpler designs we studied in the previous chapter, missing data will affect our analysis.

4.2.3. Interactions

To test the hypothesis of no interaction, we first eliminate row and column effects by subtracting the row and column means from the original observa-

---

Sidebar

Program for estimating significance level of the main effect of fertilizer on crop yield in a balanced design

Set aside space for

Monte	the number of Monte Carlo simulations
S_0	the original value of test statistic
S	test statistic for rearranged data
data	$\{5, 10, 8, 15, 22, 18, 21, 29, 25, 6, 9, 12, 25, 32, 40, 55, 60, 48\}$;
$n = 3$	number of observations in each category
blocks = 2	number of blocks
levels = 3	number of levels of factor

Main program
  Get data
    put all the observations into a single linear vector
  Compute S_0 for the original observations
  Repeat Monte times:
    for each block
      Rearrange the data in the block
    Compute S
    Compare S with S_0
  Print out the proportion of times S was larger than S_0

Rearrange
  Set s to the number of observations in the block
  Start: Choose a random integer k from 0 to $s - 1$
    Swap $X[k]$ and $X[s - 1]$:
    Decrement s and repeat from start
  Stop after you've selected all but one of the samples.

Get data
  user-written procedure gets data and packs it into a two-dimensional array in which each row corresponds to a block.

Compute
$$F1 = \sum_{i=1}^{I} \sum_{j=1}^{J} |X_{ij\cdot} - X_{\cdot j\cdot}|$$
  for each block
    calculate the mean of that block
    for each level within a block
      calculate the mean of that block-level
      calculate difference from block mean

---

tions. That is, we set

$$X'_{ijk} = X_{ijk} - X_{i\cdot\cdot} - X_{\cdot j\cdot} + X_{\cdots};$$

where by adding the grand mean, $X_{\cdots}$, we ensure the overall sum will be zero. In the example of the effect of sunlight and fertilizer on crop yield, we are left

Table 4.2. Effect of Sunlight and Fertilizer on Crop Yield. Testing for Nonadditive Interaction

S		Fertilizer		
		LO	MED	HIGH
u	LO	4.1	−2.1	−11.2
n		9.1	4.1	−3.2
l		7.1	0.1	−7.2
i				
g	HI	−9.8	−7.7	7.8
h		−6.8	−0.7	12.8
t		−3.8	7.2	0.8

with the residuals shown in Table 4.2. The pattern of plus and minus signs in this table of residuals suggests that fertilizer and sunlight affect crop yield in a superadditive fashion. Note the minus signs associated with the mismatched combinations of a high level of sunlight and a low level of fertilizer and a low level of sunlight with a high level of fertilizer. To encapsulate our intuition in numeric form, we sum the deviates within each cell, square the sum, and then sum the squares to form the test statistic

$$l = \sum_{i=1}^{I} \sum_{j=1}^{J} \left(\sum_{k=1}^{K} X'_{ijk} \right)^2$$

We compute this test statistic for each rerandomization of the 18 deviates into six subsamples. In most cases, the values of the test statistic are close to zero as the entries in each cell cancel. The value of the test statistic for our original data, $l = 2126.8$, stands out as an exceptional value and we conclude there is a significant interaction between sunlight and fertilizer ($\alpha < .003$) in addition to the separate, significant additive effects of sunlight and fertilizer.

We include our own test program as a Sidebar.

4.2.4. Designing an Experiment

All the preceding results are based on the assumption that the assignment of treatments to plots (or subjects) is made at random. While it might be convenient to fertilize our plots as shown in Figure 4.1a, the result could be a systematic bias, particularly if, for example, there is a gradient in dissolved minerals from east to west across the field.

The layout adopted in Figure 4.1b, obtained with the aid of a computerized random number generator, reduces but does not eliminate the effects of this hypothetical gradient. Because this layout was selected at random, the exchangeability of the error terms and, hence, the exactness of the cor-

---

Sidebar

Program for estimating significance level of the interaction of sunlight and
fertilizer on crop yield based on the deviates from the additive model

Set aside space for
  Monte   the number of Monte Carlo simulations
  S_0 the original value of test statistic
  S test statistic for rearranged data
  data   {5, 10, 8, 15, 22, 18, 21, 29, 25, 6, 9, 12, 25, 32, 40, 55, 60, 48};
  deviates   vector of deviates
  $n = 3$ number of observations in each category
  blocks = 2   number of blocks
  levels = 3   number of levels of factor

Main program
  Get data
  Calculate the Deviates
  Compute the test statistic S_0
  Repeat Monte times:
    Rearrange the observations
    Compute the test statistic S
    Compare S with S_0
  Print out the proportion of times S was larger than S_0

Compute

$$\sum_{i=1}^{I} \sum_{j=1}^{J} \left(\sum_{k=1}^{K} X'_{ik} \right)^2$$

  for each block
    for each level
      sum the deviates
      square this sum
      cumulate

Deviates
$X'_{ijk} = X_{ijk} - X_{i\ldots} - X_{\cdot j\cdot} + X_{\ldots}$
  Set aside space for level means, block means, and grand mean
    for each level calculate mean
    for each block
      calculate mean
      for each level
        cumulate grand mean
    for each block
      for each level
        calculate deviate from additive model

Hi	Med	Lo
Hi	Med	Lo
Hi	Med	Lo

a

Hi	Med	Lo
Lo	Lo	Med
Hi	Hi	Med

b

Hi	Med	Lo
Lo	Hi	Med
Med	Lo	Hi

c

Figure 4.1. a) Systematic assignment of fertilizer levels to plots; b) random assignment of fertilizer levels to plots; c) latin square assignment of fertilizer levels to plots.

responding permutation test is assured. Unfortunately, the layout of Figure 4.1a with its built-in bias can also result from a random assignment; its selection is neither more nor less probable than any of the other $\binom{9}{3\ 3\ 3}$ possibilities.

What can we do to avoid such an undesireable event? In the layout of Figure 4.1c, known as a Latin Square, each fertilizer level occurs once and once only in each row and in each column; if there is a systematic gradient of minerals in the soil, then this layout ensures that the gradient will have almost equal impact on each of the three treatment levels. It will have an almost equal impact even if the gradient extends from northeast to southwest rather than from east to west, or north to south. I use the phrase "almost equal" because a gradient effect may still persist. The design and analysis of Latin Squares is described in Section 4.2.7.

To increase the sensitivity of your experiments and to eliminate any systematic bias, I recommend you use the following three-step procedure during the design phase:

1) List all the factors you feel may influence the outcome of your experiment.
2) Block all factors which are under your control; this process is described in Section 3.6. You may want to use some of these factors to restrict the scope of your experiment, e.g., eliminate all individuals under 18 and over 60.

```
F                    Factor 1

a           1    2    3
c     1     A    B    C
t     2     B    C    A
o     3     C    A    B
r

2
```

Figure 4.2. A Latin Square.

3) Randomly assign units to treatment within each block. See also, Maxwell and Cole [X: 1991].[1]

4.2.5. Latin Square

The Latin Square considered in Section 4.2.5 is one of the simplest examples of an experimental design in which the statistician takes advantage of some aspect of the model to reduce the overall sample size.

A Latin Square is a three-factor experiment in which each combination of factors occurs once and once only. We can use a Latin Square as in Figure 4.2 to assess the effects of soil composition on crop yield:

In this diagram, Factor 1—gypsum concentration, for example, is increasing from left to right; Factor 2 is increasing from top to bottom (or from North to South); and the third factor, its varying levels denoted by the capital letters A, B, and C, occurs in combination with the other two in such a way that each combination of factors—row, column, and treatment—occurs once and once only.

Because of this latter restriction, there are only 12 different ways in which we can assign the varying factor levels to form a 3×3 Latin Square. Among the other 11 designs are

```
            1    2    3
      1     A    C    B
      2     B    A    C
      3     C    B    A
```

and

```
      1     C    B    A
      2     B    A    C
      3     A    C    B
```

---

[1] X preceding a date, as in Cole [X: 1991] refers to a supplemental bibliography at the end of the text which includes material not directly related to permutation methods.

Let us assume we begin our experiment by selecting one of these twelve designs at random and planting our seeds in accordance with the indicated conditions.

Because there is only a single replication of each factor combination in a Latin Square, we can not estimate the interactions. Thus, the Latin Square is appropriate *only* if we feel confident in assuming that the effects of the various factors are completely additive, that is, that the interaction terms are zero.

Our model for the Latin Square is

$$X_{ijk} = \mu + s_i + r_j + f_k + \varepsilon_{ijk}$$

where, as always in a permuation analysis, we assume that the errors ε_{ijk} are exchangeable. Our null hypothesis is $H: s_1 = s_2 = s_3$. If we assume an ordered alternative, $K: s_1 > s_2 > s_3$, our test statistic for the main effect is similar to the correlation statistic employed in equation 4.4:

$$R = \sum_{i=1}^{3} i(X_{i..} - X_{...})$$

or, equivalently, after eliminating the grand mean $X_{...}$ which is invariant under permutations,

$$R1 = \sum_{i=-1}^{1} iX_{i..} = X_{c..} - X_{A..}$$

We evaluate this test statistic both for the observed design and for each of the twelve possible Latin Square designs that might have been employed in this particular experiment. We reject the hypothesis of no treatment effect only if the test statistic for the original observations is an extreme value.

For example, suppose we employed Design 1 and observed

21	28	17
14	27	19
13	18	23

Then $3y_{A..} = 58$, $3y_{B..} = 65$, $3y_{C..} = 57$ and our test statistic $R1 = -1$. Had we employed Design 2, then $3y_{A..} = 71$, $3y_{B..} = 49$, $3y_{C..} = 65$, and our test statistic $R1 = -6$. With Design 3, $3y_{A..} = 57$, $3y_{B..} = 65$, $3y_{C..} = 58$ and our test statistic $R1 = +1$.

We see from the permutation distribution obtained in this manner that the value of our test statistic for the design actually employed in the experiment, $R1 = -1$, is an average value, not an extreme one. We accept the null hypothesis and conclude that increasing the treatment level from A to B to C does not significantly increase the yield.

4.2.6. Other Designs

If the three-step rule outlined in Section 4.2.5 leads to a more complex experimental design than those considered here, consult Kempthorne [1955]; Wilks and Kempthorne [1956, 1957]; and Scheffe [1959]. To correct for variables not under your control, see the next section.

4.3. Analysis of Covariance

4.3.1. Covariates Defined

Some variables that affect the outcome of an experiment are under our control from the very beginning—e.g., light and fertilizer. But we may only be capable of measuring rather than controlling other equally influential variables, called covariates. Blood chemistry is an example of a covariate in a biomedical experiment. Various factors in the blood can affect an experimental outcome, and most blood factors will be affected by a treatment, but few are under our direct control.

In this section, we will discuss two methods for correcting for the effects of covariates. The first, eliminating the functional relationship, is for use when you know or suspect the nature of the functional relationship between the observables and the covariates. The second method, restricted randomization, is for use when the covariates take only a few discrete values and these values can be used to restrict the randomization.

4.3.2. Eliminate the Functional Relationship

Gail, Tan, and Piantadosi [1988] recommend eliminating the effects of covariates first and then applying permutation methods to the residuals. For example, suppose the observation Y depends both on the treatment τ_i $(i = 1,\ldots,l)$ and on the p-dimensional vector of covariates $X = (X^1,\ldots,X^p)$, that is

$$Y = \mu + \tau + X\beta + e$$

where Y, μ, τ, and e are $n*1$ vectors of observations, mean values, treatment effects, and errors respectively, X is an $n*p$ matrix of covariate values, and β is a $p \times 1$ vector of regression coefficients.

We would use least squares methods to estimate the regression coefficients $\hat{\beta}$ after which we would apply the permutation methods described in the preceding sections to the residuals $Z = Y - X\hat{\beta}$.

We use a similar approach in 4.2.4 in testing a two-factor model for a significant interaction. In that example, as here, we assume that the individual errors are exchangeable. A further assumption in the present case is that both the concomitant variables (the X's) and the regression coefficients β are unaffected by the treatment [Kempthorne, 1952, p. 160].

A distribution-free multivariate analysis of covariance in which the effects of the treatments and the covariates are evaluated simultaneously is considered in the next chapter.

4.3.3. Selecting Variables

Which covariates should be included in your model? Draper and Stoneman [1966] describe a permutation procedure for selecting covariates using a *forward* stepping rule:

The first variable you select should have the largest squared sample correlation with the dependent variable y; thereafter, include the variable with the largest squared partial correlation with y given the variables that have already been selected. You may use any standard statistics package to obtain these correlations. Equivalently, you may select variables based on the maximum value of the square of the t-ratio for the regression coefficient of the entering variable, the so-called "F to enter." The problem lies in knowing when to stop, that is, in knowing when an additional variable contributes little beyond noise to the model.

Percentiles of the permutation distribution of the F-to-enter statistic can be used to test whether variables not yet added to the model would be of predictive value. Details for deriving the permutation distribution of this statistic defined in terms of Householder rotations of the permuted variable matrix are given in Forsythe et al. [1973].

4.3.4. Restricted Randomization

If the covariates take on only a few discrete values, e.g., smoker vs non-smoker, or status 0, 1, or 2 we may correct for their effects by restricting the rerandomizations to those whose design matrices match the original [Edgington, 1983].

Consider the artificial data set in Table 4.3 adapted from Rosenbaum [1984, p. 568]. To test the hypothesis that the treatment has no effect on the response, we would use the sum of the observations in the treatment group as our test statistic. The sum of 8 for the original observations is equaled or exceeded in six of the $\binom{7}{2} = 21$ possible rerandomizations. This result is not statistically significant.

Table 4.3. Data for Artificial Example

Subject	Treatment	Result	Covariate
A	1	6	1
B	1	2	0
C	0	5	1
D	0	4	1
E	0	3	1
G	0	1	0
H	0	0	0

Now let us take the covariate into consideration. One member of the original treatment group has a covariate value of 0, the other has a covariate value of 1. We limit our attention to the $12 = \binom{4}{1}\binom{3}{1}$ possible rerandomizations in which the members of the treatment group have similar covariate values. These consist of AB AG AH, CB CG CH, DB DG DH, EB EG EH. With only one of the 12, that of AB the original observations, do we observe a result sum as large as 8. This sum is statistically significant at the 0.1 level. Restricting the randomizations eliminates the masking effect of the covariate and reveals the statistically significant effect of the treatment.

If the covariate varies continuously, it may still be possible to apply the method of restricted randomizations by first subdividing the covariate's range into a few discrete categories. For example, if

$$x < -1 \quad \text{let} \quad x' = 0$$

$$-1 < x < 1 \quad \text{let} \quad x' = 1$$

$$1 < x \quad \text{let} \quad x' = 2.$$

Rosenbaum [1984] suggests that with larger samples one should restrict the randomizations so that a specific mean value of the covariate is attained, rather than a specific set of values.

Subject to certain relatively weak assumptions, the method of restricted randomizations can also be applied to after-the-fact covariates. (See Section 9.2.)

4.4. Unbalanced Designs

The permutation test is not a panacea. Imbalance in the design will result in the confounding of main effects with interactions. Consider the following two-factor model for crop yield:

$$X_{ijk} = \mu + s_i + r_j + sr_{ij} + \varepsilon_{ijk}.$$

$$N(0,1) \quad | \quad N(2,1)$$

$$N(2,1) \quad | \quad N(0,1)$$

Now suppose that the observations in a two-factor experimental design are normally distributed as in the preceding diagram taken from Cornfield and Tukey [1956]. There are no main effects in this example—both row means and both column means have the same expectations, but there is a clear interaction represented by the two nonzero off-diagonal elements.

If the design is balanced, with equal numbers per cell, the lack of significant main effects and the presence of a significant interaction should and will be confirmed by our analysis. But suppose that the design is not in balance, that for every ten observations in the first column, we have only one observation in the second. Because of this imbalance, when we use the statistic S' (equation 4.1'), we will uncover a false "row" effect which is actually due to the interaction between rows and columns. The main effect is said to be *confounded* with the interaction.

If a design is unbalanced as in the preceding example, we cannot test for a "pure" main effect or a "pure" interaction. But we may be able to test for the combination of a main effect with an interaction by using the statistic (S', $F1'$ or R') that we would use to test for the main effect alone. This combined effect will not be confounded with the main effects of other unrelated factors.

For 3-factor designs with unequal sample sizes, the test statistics for mixed main/interaction effects are:

$$S' = \sum_{j=1}^{J} \sum_{k=1}^{K} \sum_{1=m_{jk}+1}^{(n_{jk}+m_{jk})} X_{jkl} \tag{4.1'}$$

$$F1' = \sum_{j=1}^{J} \sum_{k=1}^{K} \sum_{i=1}^{I} n_{ijk} |X_{ijk\cdot} - X_{\cdot jk\cdot}| \tag{4.3'}$$

$$R' = \sum_{j=1}^{J} \sum_{k=1}^{K} \sum_{i=1}^{I} f[i] n_{ijk} (X_{ijk\cdot} - X_{\cdot jk\cdot}) \tag{4.4'}$$

4.4.1. Missing Combinations

If an entire factor-combination is missing, we may not be able to estimate or test any of the effects. One very concrete example is an unbalanced design I encountered in the 1970's:

Makinodan et al. [1976] studied the effects of age on the mediation of the immune response. They measured the anti-SBRC response of spleen cells derived from C57BL mice of various ages. In one set of trials, the cells were derived entirely from the spleens of young mice, in a second set of trials, they came from the spleens of old mice, and in a third they came from mixtures of the two.

Let $X_{i,j,k}$ denote the response of the kth sample taken from a population of type i, j ($i = 0 = j$: controls; $i = 1$, $j = 0$: cells from young animals only; $i = 0, j = 1$: cells from old animals only; $i = 1 = j$: mixture of cells from old and young animals.) We assume that for lymphocytes taken from the spleens of young animals,

$$X_{2,1,k} = \mu + \alpha + e_{2,1,k},$$

for the spleens of old animals,

$$X_{1,2,k} = \mu - \alpha + e_{1,2,k},$$

and for a mixture of p spleens from young animals and $(1 - p)$ spleens from old animals, where $0 \le p \le 1$,

$$X_{2,2,k} = p(\mu + \alpha) + (1 - p)(\mu - \alpha) - \gamma + e_{2,2,k}$$
$$= \mu + (1 - 2p)\alpha - \gamma + e_{2,2,k},$$

where the $e_{i,j,k}$ are independent values.

Makinodan knew in advance of his experiment that $\alpha > 0$. He also knew that the distributions of the errors $e_{i,j,k}$ would be different for the different populations. We can assume only that these errors are independent of one another and that their medians are zero.

Makinodan wanted to test the hypothesis $\gamma = 0$ as there are immediate biological interpretations for the three alternatives: from $\gamma = 0$ one may infer independent action of the two cell populations; $\gamma < 0$ means excess lymphocytes in young populations; and $\gamma > 0$ suggests the presence of suppressor cells in the spleens of older animals.

But what statistic are we to use to do the test? One possibility is

$$S = |X_{2,2,.} - pX_{1,2,.} - (1 - p)X_{2,1,.}|.$$

If the design were balanced, or we could be sure that the null effect $\mu = 0$, this is the statistic we would use. But the design is not balanced, with the result that the main effects (in which we are not interested) are confounded with the interaction (in which we are).

It is small consolation that the standard parametric (ANOVA) approach won't work in this example either. Fortunately, another resampling method, the bootstrap, can provide a solution.

Here is the bootstrap procedure:

Draw an observation at random and with replacement from the set $\{x_{2,1,k}\}$; label it $x_{2,1,j}^*$. Similarly, draw the bootstrap observations $x_{1,2,j}^*$ and $x_{2,2,j}^*$ from the sets $\{x_{1,2,k}\}$ and $\{x_{2,2,k}\}$.

Let $\quad z_j = px_{1,2,j}^* + (1 - p)x_{2,1,j}^* - x_{2,2,j}^*.$

Repeat this resampling procedure a thousand or more times, obtaining a bootstrap estimate z_j of the interaction each time you resample. Use the resultant set of bootstrap estimates $\{z_j\}$ to obtain a confidence interval for γ. If 0 belongs to this confidence interval, accept the hypothesis of additivity; otherwise reject.

One word of caution: unlike a permutation test, a bootstrap is exact only for very large samples. The probability of a Type I error may be greater than the significance level you specify.

Sidebar

Mean DPFC response. Effect of pooled old BC3FL spleen cells on the anti-SRBC response of indicator pooled BC3FL spleen cells. Data extracted from Makinodan et al (1976). Bootstrap analysis.

Young Cells	Old Cells	1/2 + 1/2
5640	1150	7100
5120	2520	11020
5780	900	13065
4430	50	
7230		

Bootstrap sample 1:	5640 + 900 − 11020	−4480
Bootstrap sample 2:	5780 + 1150 − 11020	−4090
Bootstrap sample 2:	7230 + 1150 − 7100	1280
. . . .	. . . .	. .
. . . .	. . . .	. .
Bootstrap sample 600:	5780 + 2520 − 7100	1200

4.5. Clinical Trials

4.5.1. Avoiding Unbalanced Designs

In preceding sections, we tacitly assumed that the assignment of subjects to treatment took place *before* the start of the experiment. We also assumed, tacitly, that the assignment of subjects to treatment was *double blind*, that is, neither the experimental subject nor the experimenter knew which treatment the subject was receiving. (See Fisher [1935] and Feinstein [1981] for a justification of this double blind approach.) But in a large clinical trial covering several hundreds, even thousands of patients in various treatment categories, not all of the subjects will be available prior to the start of treatment. We even may have tabulated some of the results before the last of the patients have enrolled in the experiment. If we let pure chance determine whether an incoming patient is assigned to treatment or control, the trials may quickly go out of balance and stay out of balance. On the other hand, if we insist on keeping the experiment balanced at each stage, assigning subjects alternately to treatment and placebo, a physician could crack the code, guesstimate the next treatment assignment, and be influenced in her handling of a patient as a result.

One solution [Efron, X: 1971] is to weight the probability of a particular treatment assignment in accordance with the assignments that have already taken place. For example, if the last subject was assigned to the control group, we might increase the probability of assigning the current subject to the treatment from $\frac{1}{2}$ to $\frac{3}{4}$. The assignment is still random—so no one can crack the code, but there will be a tendency for the two groups—treatment and control—to even out in size. Of course, Efron's biased coin approach is only one of many possible restricted designs. A general form is provided in Smith [X: 1984].

While the numbers of subjects in the various treatment groups will (in theory) even out in the long run, in most cases they will still be unequal when the experiment is completed, taking values $\{n_i, i = 1, \ldots, l\}$. Fortunately, we may analyze this experiment as if these were the sample sizes we had intended from the very beginning [Cox, 1982].

Following Hollander and Pena [1988], suppose there are R possible treatments. Let $T_j = (T_{j1}, \ldots, T_{jR-1})'$ be the treatment assignment vector for the jth patient; $j = 1, \ldots, n$. T_{ji} is equal to 1 or 0 according to whether patient j is or is not assigned to treatment i. Let $x_n = (x_1, \ldots, x_n)'$ be the vector of patient responses (e.g., time to death, time to relapse). We want to test the null hypothesis that the R treatments are equivalent. The randomization distribution of the test statistic $S_n = (T_1, \ldots, T_n)x_n$ induced by the randomized treatment allocation grows increasingly more complicated with increasing n. Nevertheless, it may be determined by recursive means.

Smith and Wei [1983] show that the permutation method can provide an exact test in the case of two treatments. Their result is extended to k-treatments by Wei, Smythe, and Smith [1986]. Algorithms for computing the exact distribution of the test statistic, rather than an asymptotic approximation, are provided by Hollander and Pena [1988] and Mehta, Patel, and Wei [1988].

4.5.2. Missing Data

A further and as yet unresolved problem in the analysis of clinical trials is the dropping out of patients during the course of the investigation. When such dropouts occur at random, we still may apply any of the standard permutation methods, that is if we are prepared to deal with confounded effects (see Section 4.5). But what if the dropout rate is directly related to the treatment! In a study of a medication guaranteed to lower cholesterol levels in the blood, a midwest pharmaceutical company found itself without any patients remaining in the treatment group. The medicine, alas, tasted too much like sand coated with slimy egg whites and chalk dust.

In several less extreme cases, Entsuah [1990] shows that permutation methods can be applied even if withdrawal is related to treatment, providing we modify our scoring system to account for the dropouts. Entsuah studies and compares the power of scoring systems based on functions of boundaries, endpoints, and time using either the ranks or the original observations. His results are specific to the applications he studied.

4.6. Very Large and Very Small Samples

When the sample sizes are very large, from several dozen to several hundred observations per group, as they often are in clinical trials, the time required to compute a permutation distribution can be prohibitive even if we are taking advantage of one of the optimal computing algorithms described in Chapter 13. Fortunately, when sample sizes are large—and we refer here to the size of the smallest sub-sample corresponding to a specific factor combination, not to the size of the sample as a whole, we can make use of an asymptotic approximation in place of the exact permutation distribution. A series of papers by Hoeffding [1951], Box and Anderson [1955], and Kempthorne et al. [1961] support the replacement of the permutation distribution of the F-statistic by the tabulated distribution of the F-ratio. This approximation can often be improved on if we replace the observed values by their corresponding ranks or normal scores. Sections 9.3 and 14.3 provide additional discussion of these points.

With very small samples, the permutation distribution is readily calculated. But with few observations, the power of the test may well be too small and we run the risk of overlooking a treatment effect that is of practical significance. A solution in some cases is to take our observations in stages, rejecting or accepting the null hypothesis at each stage only if the p-value of the data is very large or very small. Otherwise, we continue to take more observations.

4.7. Questions

1. Rewrite the computer program in Section 4.2.3 so it will yield the permutation distributions of the three k-sample statistics. $F1$, $F2$, and R. Would you still accept/reject the hypothesis if you used $F2$ or R in place of $F1$?

2. *Confidence interval.* Derive a 90% confidence interval for the main effect of sunlight using the crop yield data in Table 4.1. First, restate the model so as to make clear what it is you are estimating:

$$X_{ikl} = \mu + s_i + f_k + sf_{ik} + \varepsilon_{ikl},$$

$$\text{with} \quad s_1 = -\delta \quad \text{and} \quad s_2 = \delta.$$

Recall that we rejected the null hypothesis that $\delta = 0$. Suppose you add $d = 1$ to each of the observations in the low sunlight group and subtract $d = 1$ from each of the observations in the high sunlight group. Would you still reject the null hypothesis at the 90% level? If your answer is "yes" then $d = 1$ does not belong to the 90% confidence interval for δ. If your answer is "no" then $d = 1$ does belong. Experiment (be systematic) until you find a value δ_0 such that you accept the null hypothesis whenever $d > \delta_0$.

3. *Covariate analysis.* Suppose your observations obey the model:

$$Y_{ik} = \mu + s_i + bX_k + \varepsilon_{ik},$$

where the errors ε_{ik} are exchangeable. What statistic would you use to test if $b = 0$? to test that $s_i = 0$ for all i?

4. Equality of the slopes of two lines. Suppose you observed samples from two populations and that

$$Y_{1k} = \mu_1 + b_1 X_k + \varepsilon_{1k},$$

$$Y_{2k} = \mu_2 + b_2 X_k + \varepsilon_{ik},$$

where the errors ε_{ik} are exchangeable. What statistic would you use to test that $b_1 = b_2$, that is, that the effect of X on Y is the same in the two populations? See Chapter 7.

5. Design an experiment. a) List all the factors that might influence the outcome of your experiment. b) Write a model in terms of these factors. c) Which factors are under your control? d) Which of these factors will you use to restrict the scope of the experiment? e) Which of these factors will you use to block? f) Which of the remaining factors will you neglect initially, that is, lump into your error term? g) How will you deal with each of the remaining covariates? h) By correction? i) By blocking after the fact? j) How many subjects will you observe in each subcategory? k) Is the subject the correct experimental unit? l) Write out two of the possible assignments of subjects to treatment. m) How many possible assignments are there in all?

CHAPTER 5

Multivariate Analysis

5.1. Introduction

The value of an analysis based on simultaneous observations on several variables—height, weight, blood pressure, and cholesterol level, for example, is that it can be used to detect subtle changes that might not be detectable, except with very large, prohibitively expensive samples, were you to consider only one variable at a time.

Any of the permutation procedures described in Chapters 3 and 4 can be applied in a multivariate setting providing we can find a single-valued test statistic which can stand in place of the multivalued vector of observations.

5.2. One- and Two-Sample Comparisons

5.2.1. Hotelling's T^2

One example of such a statistic is Hotelling's T^2, a straightforward generalization of Student's t to the multivariate case.

Suppose we have made a series of exchangeable vector-valued observations $\vec{X}_i = \{X_{i1}, X_{i2}, \dots, X_{iJ}\}$, for $i = 1, \dots, I$. Let $\vec{X}.$ denote the vector of mean values $\{X._1, X._2, \dots, X._J\}$, and V the $J \times J$ covariance matrix; that is, V_{ij} is the covariance of X_{ki} and X_{kj}. To test the hypothesis that the midvalue of $\vec{X}_i = \vec{\xi}$ for all i, use

$$\text{Hotelling's } T^2 = (\vec{X}. - \vec{\xi})V^{-1}(\vec{X}. - \vec{\xi})^T.$$

Loosely speaking, this statistic weighs the contribution of individual variables and pairs of variables in inverse proportion to their covariances. If the variables in each observation vector are independent of one another (a rare case, indeed), Hotelling's T^2 weighs the contributions of the individual variables in inverse proportion to their variances.

The two-sample comparison is only slightly more complicated: Let n_1, $\vec{X}_1.; n_2, \vec{X}_2.$ denote the sample size and vector of mean values of the first and second samples respectively. We assume under the null hypothesis that the two sets of vector-valued observations $\{\vec{X}_{1i}\}$ and $\{\vec{X}_{2i}\}$ come from the same distribution (that is, the sample labels 1 and 2 are exchangeable). Let V denote the pooled estimate of the common covariance matrix; as in the one-sample case, V_{ij} denotes the pooled covariance estimate of X_{1ki} and X_{2kj},

$$(N - 2)V_{ij} = \sum_{m=1}^{2} \sum_{k=1}^{n_i} (X_{mki} - X_{..i})(X_{mkj} - X_{..j})$$

To test the hypothesis that the midvalues of the two distributions are the same, we could use the statistic

$$T^2 = (\vec{X}_1. - \vec{X}_2.)V^{-1}(\vec{X}_1. - \vec{X}_2.)^T.$$

but then we would be forced to recompute the covariance matrix V and its inverse V^{-1} for each new rearrangement. To reduce the number of computations, Wald and Wolfowitz [1943] suggest a slightly different statistic T' that is a monotonic function of T (see Problem 3).
    Let

$$U_j = N^{-1} \sum_{i=1}^{2} \sum_{k=1}^{n_i} X_{ikj}$$

$$c_{ij} = \sum_{m=1}^{2} \sum_{k=1}^{n_i} (X_{mki} - U_i)(X_{mkj} - U_j)$$

Let C be the matrix whose components are the c_{ij}. Then

$$T'^2 = (\vec{X}_1. - \vec{X}_2.)C^{-1}(\vec{X}_1. - \vec{X}_2.)^T.$$

As with all permutation tests we proceed in three steps:

(1) we compute the test statistic for the original observations;
(2) we compute the test statistic for all relabelings;
(3) we determine the percentage of relabelings that lead to values of the test statistic that are as extreme or more extreme than the orginal value.

For the purpose of relabeling, each vector of observations on an individual subject is treated as a single indivisible entity. When we relabel, we relabel on a subject-by-subject basis so that all observations on a single subject receive the same new label. If the original vector of observations on subject i consists of k distinct observations on k different variables

$$(x_i^1, x_i^2, \ldots, x_i^k)$$

and we give this vector a new label $p(i)$, then the individual observations remain together as a unit, each with the new label:

Sidebar

Calculating the Wald-Wolfowitz variant of Hotelling's T^2 Blood Chemistry Data from Warner et al. [X: 1990]

ID	BC	Albumin	Uric Acid			
2381	N	43	54	Mean	Albumin	Uric Acid
1610	N	41	33	N	41.25	46.25
1149	N	39	50	Y	37.0	52.75
2271	N	42	48	Comb	39.125	49.5
				Y−N	−4.25	6.50
1946	Y	35	72	C		
1797	Y	38	30			
575	Y	40	46		8.982	−21.071
39	Y	35	63		−21.071	196.571
				C^{-1}		
					.1487	.01594
					.01594	.006796

Hotelling's T^2

$$= (-4.25 \ \ 6.50)C^{-1}(-4.25 \ \ 6.50)^T$$
$$= 2.092$$

$$(x^1_{p(i)}, x^2_{p(i)}, \ldots, x^k_{p(i)})$$

This approach to relabeling should be contrasted with the approach we would use if we were testing for independence of the covariates (see Section 7.1).

Hotelling's T^2 is the appropriate statistic to use if you suspect the data has a distribution that is close to that of the multivariate normal. Under the assumption of multivariate normality, the power of the permutation version of Hotelling's T^2 converges with increasing sample size to the power of the most powerful parametric test that is invariant under transformations of scale.

The stated significance level of the parametric version of Hotelling's T^2 can not be relied on for small samples if the data is not normally distributed [Davis, X: 1982][1]. As always, the corresponding permutation test yields an exact significance level even if the errors are not normally distributed, providing that the errors are exchangeable from sample to sample.

Much of the theoretical work on Hotelling's T^2 has focused on the properties of the *unconditional*[2] permutation test in which the original observations are replaced by ranks. Details of the asymptotic properties and power of the

---

[1] X preceding a date, as in Davis [X: 1982] refers to a supplemental bibliography at the end of the text which includes material not directly related to permutation methods.

[2] Recall from our discussion in Section 2.3 that whereas we must compute the permutation distribution anew for each new set of observations, the permutation distribution of a set of ranks is independent or unconditional of the actual values of the observations.

unconditional test are given in Barton and David [1961], Chatterjee and Sen [1964, 1966], and, most recently, Gill and Siotani [1987]. The effect of missing observations on the significance level and power of the test is studied by Servy and Sen [1987].

5.2.2. An Example

The following blood chemistry data is taken from Werner et al. [X: 1970]. The full data set is included with the BMDP statistical package. An asterisk (*) denotes missing data.

1	2	3	4	5	6	7	8	9
2381	22	67	144	N	200	43	98	54
1946	22	64	160	Y	600	35	*	72
1610	25	62	128	N	243	41	104	33
1797	25	68	150	Y	50	38	96	30
1149	53	*	178	N	227	39	*	50
575	53	65	140	Y	220	40	107	46
2271	54	66	158	N	305	42	103	48
39	54	60	170	Y	220	35	88	63

The variables are

1. identification number
2. age in years
3. height in inches
4. weight in pounds
5. uses birth control pills?
6. cholesterol level
7. albumin level
8. calcium level
9. uric acid level

A potential hypothesis of interest is whether birth control usage has any effect on blood chemistries. As the nature of such hypothetical effects very likely depends upon age and years of use, before testing this hypothesis using a permutation method, you might want to divide the data into two blocks corresponding to young and old patients.

You could test several univariate hypotheses using the methods of Section 3.5; for example—the hypothesis that using birth control pills lowers the albumin level in blood. You might want to do this now to see if you can obtain significant results. As the sample sizes are small, the univariate observations may not be statistically significant. But by combining the observations that Warner and his colleagues made on several different variables to form a single multivariate statistic, you may obtain a statistically significant result; that is, if taking birth control pills does alter blood chemistries.

Sidebar

Program for computing multivariate permutation statistics
define length   119
define control   60
define variates   9

Set aside space for a multivariate array Data [length, variates]; and a vector of
    sample sizes index[length];

Main program
  Load (Data);
  Compute stat0 (Data, index);
  repeat Nsim times
    Rearrange Data;
    Compute stat (Data, index);
    record whether stat $>=$ stat0;
  print out the significance level of the test

Load
  packs the data into a long matrix each row of which corresponds to k observations on a single subject; the first n rows are the control group; the last m rows
  are the treatment group. (a second use of this subroutine will be to eliminate
  variables and subjects that will not be included in the analysis, e.g., to eliminate
  all records that include missing data, and to define and select specific subgroups.)

Rearrange
  randomly rearranges the rows of the Data array; the elements in each row are
  left in the same order.

Compute
  calculate the mean of each variable for each sample and store the results in a
    2 by n array N;
  calculate n by n array V of covariances for the combined sample and invert V;
  matrix mult (Mean, W, *W);
  matrix mult (W, Mean);
  return T'^2

5.2.3. Doing the Computations

You don't need to use all the dependent variables in forming Hotelling's T^2. For example, you could just include albumin and uric acid levels as we have in a sidebar. For each relabeling, you would need to compute four sample means corresponding to the two variables and the two treatment groups. And you would need to perform two successive matrix multiplications. I would not attempt these calculations without a computer and the appropriate computer software: Warner et al.'s full data set includes 188 cases!

As in the univariate examples in Chapters 3 and 4, you need to program and implement three procedures:

a) one to rearrange the stored data;
b) one to compute the T^2 statistic;
c) and one to compute the significance level.

Only the first of these procedures, devoted to rearranging the data, represents a significant change from the simple calculations we performed in the univariate case. In a multivariate analysis, we can't afford to manipulate the actual data; a simple swap could mean the exchange of nine or ten or even a hundred different variables; so we rearrange a vector of indices that point to the data instead. Here is a fragment of code in the C programming language that does just that:

```
float Data [length, variates];
int index[length];
....
rearrange (index, length);
....
for (j = 0; < ncontrol; j++) Mean [k] + = Data [index[j], k];
```

5.2.4. Weighting the Variables

With several variables simultaneously lending their support to (or withholding their support from) a hypothesis or an alternative, should some variables be given more weight than others? Or should all variables be given the same importance?

In any multivariate application, whether or not you use Hotelling's T^2 as the test statistic, you may want to "Studentize" the variables by dividing by the covariance matrix before you begin.

Hotelling's T^2 Studentizes the variables in the sense that it weights each variable in inverse proportion to its standard deviation. (This is not quite true if the variables are correlated; see below.) As a result, Hotelling's T^2 is dimensionless; it will not matter if we express a vector of measurements in feet rather than inches or miles. Variables whose values fluctuate widely from observation to observation are given less weight than variables whose values are essentially constant.

When we convert an observation on a variable to the corresponding rank or normal score (see Section 9.2), we are also standardizing it. If we have exactly the same number of observations on each variable—as would be the case, for example, if all the observations on all the variables have been accurately recorded and none are missing, then all ranked variables will have exactly the same variance. The problem of what emphasis to give each individual variable is solved automatically.

Although we have standardized the variances in forming a rank test, we must still divide by the covariances. When we divide by the covariance or, equivalently in the case of ranks, by the correlation, we are discounting the importance and reducing the effects of *correlated* or dependent variables. If we have two perfectly-correlated variables—the testimony of a ventriloquist and his dummy, say, then, clearly the second variable (or witness) has no information to contribute beyond that which we have already received from the first.

5.2.5. Interpreting the Results

The significance of T^2 or some equivalent multivariate statistic still leaves unanswered the question of *which* variables have led to the rejection of the multivariate hypothesis. For a discussion of the problem of simultaneous inference, see any text on multivariate methods, for example, Morrison [X: 1990]. My own preference on finding a significant result, a preference that reflects my studies under Jerzy Neyman, is to search for a mechanistic, cause-and-effect model that will explain the findings. In Chapters 7 through 10, we consider some of the tests one might perform to verify or disprove such a model.

5.2.6. Alternative Statistics

Hotelling's T^2 is designed to test the null hypothesis of no difference between the distributions of the treated and untreated groups against alternatives that involve a shift of the k-dimensional center of the multivariate distribution. Although Hotelling's T^2 offers protection against a wide variety of alternatives, it is not particularly sensitive to alternatives that entail a shift in just one of the dependent variables.

Boyett and Shuster [1977] show that a more powerful test against such alternatives is based on the permutation distribution of the test statistic

$$\max_{1 \le k \le k} \frac{(X_1^k. - X_2^k.)}{SE^k}$$

a statistic first proposed in a permutation context by Chung and Fraser [1958], where SE^k is a pooled estimate of the standard error of the mean of the kth variable.

Let us apply this approach to the subsample of blood chemistry data we studied in Section 5.2.1. We use a two-sided test so we may detect changes up or down. For albumin, the absolute difference in means is 4.25 and the standard error is $\sqrt{8.982/2} = 1.498$; for uric acid, the difference is 6.5, the standard error is 7.010. Our test statistic is 2.84, the larger of the two weighted differences. To determine whether this value is significant, we need to compute the sample means, their differences, and the maximum difference after weighting by our estimates of the standard errors for each of the $\binom{8}{4} = 70$ rearrangements of the two samples.

5.3. Runs Test

Friedman and Rafesky [1979] provide a multivariate generalization of the Wald-Wolfowitz and Smirnov distribution-free two-sample tests used for testing $F_X = F_Y$ against the highly nonspecific alternative $F_X \neq F_Y$. In both the univariate and the multivariate versions of these two-sample tests, one measures the degree to which the two samples are segregated within the combined sample. In the univariate version, one forms a single combined sample, sorts and orders it, and then

a) counts the number of runs in the combined sample; or
b) computes the maximum difference in cumulative frequency of the two types within the combined sample.

For example if $x = (1, 3, 6)$ and $y = (2, 4, 5)$, the ordered combined sample is 1, 2, 3, 4, 5, 6, that is, an x followed by $y \times yy \times$, and has five runs.

Highly segregated samples will give rise to a small number of runs (and a large maximum difference in cumulative frequency), while highly interlaced distributions will give rise to a large number of runs (and a very small difference in cumulative frequency). Statistical significance, that is, whether the number of runs is significantly large, can be determined from the permutation distribution of the test statistic.

To create a multivariate version of these tests, we must find a way to order observations that have multiple coordinates. The key to this ordering is the *minimal spanning tree* described by Friedman and Rafesky [1979]:

Each point in Figure 5.1A corresponds to a pair of observations, e.g. height and weight, that were made on a single subject. We build a spanning tree between these data points as in Figure 5.1B, by connecting the points so that there is exactly one path between each pair of points, and so that no path closes back on itself in a loop. Obviously, we could construct a large number of such trees. A minimal spanning tree is one for which the sum of the lengths of all the paths is a minimum. This tree is unique if there are no ties among the $N(N-1)/2$ interpoint distances.

Before computing the test statistic(s) in the multivariate case, we first construct the minimal spanning tree for the combined sample. Once the tree is complete, we can generate the permutation distribution of the runs statistic through a series of random relabelings of the individual data points. After each relabelling, we remove all edges for which the defining nodes originate from different samples. Figure 5.1C illustrates one such result.

Although it can take a multiple of $N \times N$ calculations to construct the minimal spanning tree for a sample of size N, each determination of the multivariate runs statistic only takes a multiple of N calculations. For large samples a normal approximation to the permutation distribution may be used (see Section 12.5); the expected value and variance of the runs statistic are the same as in the univariate case.

5.3.1. Which Statistic?

We've now considered three multivariate test statistics for testing hypothesis based on one or two samples. Which one should we use? To detect a simultaneous shift in the means of several variables, use Hotelling's T^2; to detect a shift in *any* of several variables, use the maximum t; and to detect an arbitrary change in a distribution (not necessarily a shift) use Friedman and Rafesky's multivariate runs test.

Tests proposed by van-Putten [1987] and Henze [1988] offer advantages over Friedman-Rafesky in some cases.

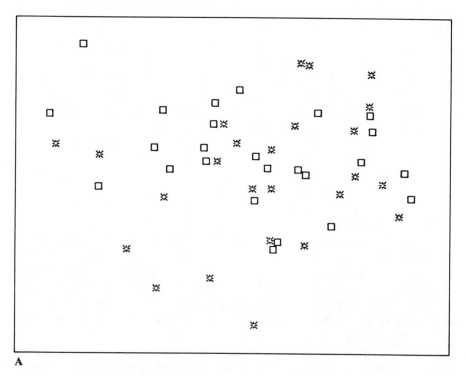

A

Figure 5.1. Building a minimal spanning tree.
From "Multivariate generalizations of the Wald–Wolfowitz and Smirnov two-sample test," by J.H. Friedman and L.C. Rafsky, *Annals of Statistics*; 1979; 7: 697–717. Reprinted with permission from the Institute of Mathematical Statistics.
    Continued next page.

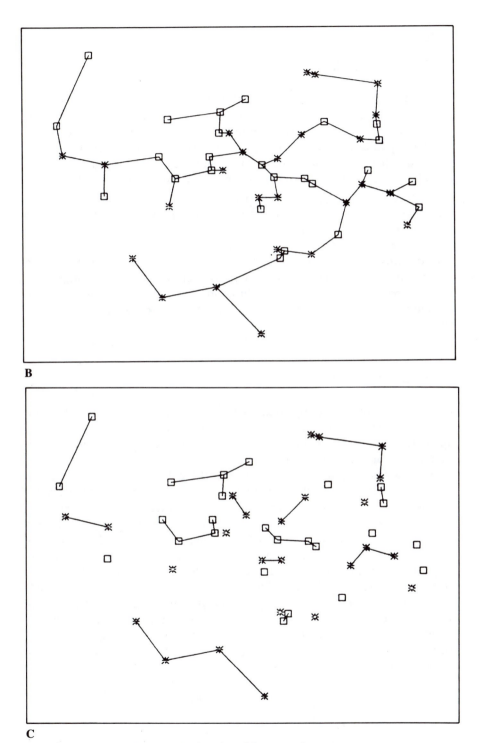

B

C

Figure 5.1. Continued from previous page.

5.4. Experimental Designs

5.4.1. Matched Pairs

Puri and Shane [1970] study the multivariate generalization of paired comparisons in an incomplete blocks design (see Sections 3.6 and 3.7). Their procedure is a straightforward generalization of the multivariate one-sample test developed by Sen and Puri [1967]; (see also Sen [1967, 1969]).

For simplicity, suppose we have only a single block. As in Section 3.1, we consider all possible permutations of the signs of the individual multivariate observations. If $\{\vec{X}_i, \vec{Y}_i\}$ is the p-dimensional vector of observations on the ith matched pair, and $\vec{Z}_i$ is the vector of differences $(Z^1, \ldots, Z^p)$, then our permutation set consists of vectors of differences of the form $((-1)^{j_1} Z_1, \ldots, (-1)^{j_n} Z_n)$ where $-Z = (-Z^1, \ldots, -Z^p)$.

Depending on the hypothesis and alternatives of interest, one may want to apply an initial set of linear transformations to each separate coordinate, that is, to replace Z^j by $Z^{\cdot j} = a_j + b_j Z^j$. Puri and Shane studied the case in which the individual variables were replaced by their ranks, with each variable being ranked separately.

5.4.2. Block Effects

When we have more than two treatments to compare, an alternative statistic studied by Gerig [1969] is the multivariate extension of Friedman's chi-square test in which ranks take the place of the original observations creating an unconditional permutation test.

The experimental units are divided into B blocks each of size I with the elements of each block as closely matched as possible with respect to extraneous variables. During the design phase, one individual from each block is assigned to each of the I treatments. We assume that K (possibly) dependent observations are made simultaneously on each subject. To test the hypothesis of identical treatment effects against translation-type alternatives, we first rank each individual variable separately within each block, ranking them from 1 to I (smallest to largest). The rank totals $T_{\cdot i(k)}$ are computed for each treatment i and each variable (k). The use of ranks automatically rescales each variable so that the variances (but not the covariances) are the same.

Let T denote the $I \times K$ matrix whose ikth component is $T_{\cdot i(k)}$. Noting that the expected value of $T_{\cdot i(k)}$ is $(K + 1)/2$, let V denote the matrix whose components are the sample covariances

$$V_{st} = \frac{\left[\sum_{b=1}^{B} \sum_{i=1}^{I} T_{bi(s)} T_{bi(t)} - \frac{k(k+1)^2}{4} \right]}{n(k-1)}.$$

By analogy with Hotelling's T^2, the test statistic is $TV^{-1}T^T$ [Gerig, 1969]. Gerig [1975] extends these results to include and correct for random covariates.

5.5. Repeated Measures

In many experiments, we want to study the development of a process over a period of time, such as the growth of a tumor or the gradual progress of a cure. If our observations are made by sacrificing different groups of animals at different periods of time, then time is simply another variable in the analysis which we may treat as a covariate. But if all our observations are made on the same subjects, then the multiple observations on a single individual will be interdependent. And all the observations on a single subject must be treated as a single multivariate vector.

We may ask at least three questions about the response profiles: (1) Are the response profiles the same for the various treatments? (2) Are the response profiles parallel? (3) Are the response profiles at the same level?

A "yes" answer to question 1 implies "yes" answers to questions (2) and (3), but we may get a "yes" answer to 2 even when the answer to (3) is "no".

One simple test of parallelism entails computing the successive differences $z_{j,i} = x_{j,i+1} - x_{j,i}$ for $j = 1, 2; i = 1, \ldots, l - 1$ and then applying the methods from Sections 5.2 or 5.3 to these differences. Of course, this approach is applicable only if the observations on both treatments were made at identical times.

To circumvent this limitation and to obtain a test of the narrower hypothesis (1), we follow Koziol et al. [1981] and suppose there are N_i subjects in group i. Let X^i_{tj}, $t = 1, 2, \ldots, T$; and $j = 1, 2, \ldots, N_i$ denote the observation on the jth subject in Group i at time t. Not all the X^i_{tj} may be observed in practice; we will only have observations for N_{it} of the N_i in the ith group at time t. If X^i_{tj} is observed, let R^i_{tj} be its rank among the $N._t$ available values at time t. Set $S_{it} = (N_{it})^{-1} \sum R_{tj}$.

If luck is with us so that all subjects remain with us to the end of the experiment, then $N_{it} = N_i$ for all t and each i, and we may adopt as our test statistic $L_N = \sum N_i \vec{S}_i^T V^{-1} \vec{S}_i$, where $\vec{S}_i$ is a $T \times 1$ vector with components $(S_{i1}, S_{i2}, \ldots, S_{iT})$ and V is a $T \times T$ covariance matrix whose stth component

$$v_{st} = N^{-1} \sum_{i=1}^{I} \sum_{j=1}^{N_i} R^i_{sj} R^i_{tj}.$$

This test statistic was proposed and investigated by Puri and Sen [1966, 1969, 1971].

5.5.1. Missing Data

If we are missing data, and missing data is almost inevitable in any large clinical study since individuals commonly postpone or even skip follow-up appointments, then no such simplified statistic presents itself. Zerbe and Walker [1977] suggest that each subject's measurements first be reduced to a vector of polynomial regression coefficients with time the independent variable. The subjects needn't have been measured at identical times or over identical periods, nor does each subject need to have the same number of observations. Only the number of coefficients (the rank of the polynomial), needs to be the same for each subject. Thus, we may apply the equations of Koziol et al. to these vectors of coefficients though we can not apply the equations to the original data.

We replace the m_k observations on the kth subject, $\{X_{ki}, i = 1, \ldots, m_k\}$ with a set of $J + 1$ coefficients, $\{b_{kj}, j = 0, \ldots, J\}$. While the m_k may vary, the number J is the same for every subject; of course, $J < m_k$ for all k. The $\{b_{kj}\}$ are chosen so that for all k and i,

$$X_{ki} \doteq b_{k0} + t_{ki}b_{ki} + \cdots + t_{ki}^{J}b_{kJ},$$

where the $\{t_{ki}, i = 0, \ldots, m_k\}$ are the observation times for the kth subject.

This approach has been adopted by a number of practitioners including Albert et al. [1982], Chapelle et al. [1982], Goldberg et al. [1980], and Hiatt et al. [1983]. Multiple comparison procedures based on it include Foutz et al. [1985] and Zerbe and Murphy [1986]. A SAS/IML program to do the calculations is available [P: Nelson and Zerbe, 1988][1].

5.5.2. Bioequivalence

Zerbe and Walker's solution to the problem of missing data suggests a multivariate approach we may use with any time course data. For example, when we do a bioequivalence study, we replace a set of discrete values with a "smooth" curve. This curve is derived in one of two ways: 1) by numerical analysis, 2) by modelling. The first yields a set of coefficients, the second a set of parameter estimates. Either the coefficients or the estimates may be treated as if they were the components of a multivariate vector and the methods of this chapter applied to them.

Here is an elementary example: Suppose you observe the time course of a drug in the urine over a period for which a linear model would be appropriate. Suppose further that the chief virtue of your measuring system is its low cost; the individual measurements are crude and imprecise. To gain precision, you take a series of measurements on each patient about half an hour apart

---

[1] The P preceding a date, as in March, P: 1972, refers to a separate bibliography at the end of the text devoted exclusively to computational methods.

and use least squares methods to derive a best-fitting line for each patient. That is, you replace the set of measurements $\{X_{ijk}\}$ where $i = 0$ or 1 denotes the drug, $j = 1, \ldots, J$ denotes the subject, and $k = 1, \ldots, K_j$ denotes the observation on a subject, with the set of vectors $\{\overline{Y}_{ij} = (a_{ij}, b_{ij})\}$ where a_{ij} and b_{ij} are the intercept and slope of the regression line for the jth subject in the ith treatment group.

Using the computer code in Section 5.2, you calculate the mean vector and the covariance matrix for the $\{\overline{Y}_{ij}\}$, and compute Hotelling's T^2 for the original observations and for a set of random arrangements. You use the resultant permutation distribution to determine whether the time courses of the two drugs are similar.

5.6. Questions

1. You can increase the power of a statistical test in three ways: a) making additional observations, b) making more precise observations, c) adding covariates. Discuss this remark in the light of your own experimental efforts.

2. You are studying a new tranquilizer which you hope will minimize the effects of stress. The peak effects of stress manifest themselves between five and ten minutes after the stressful incident, depending on the individual. To be on the safe side, you've made observations at both the five- and ten-minute marks.

Subject	pre-stress	5-minute	10-minute	Treatment
A	9.3	11.7	10.5	Brand A
B	8.4	10.0	10.5	Brand A
C	7.8	10.4	9.0	Brand A
D	7.5	9.2	9.0	New drug
E	8.9	9.5	10.2	New drug
F	8.3	9.5	9.5	New drug

How would you correct for the pre-stress readings? Is this a univariate or a multivariate problem? List possible univariate and multivariate test statistics. Perform the permutation tests and compare the results.

3. Show that if T' is a monotonic function of T, then a test based on the permutation distribution of T' will accept or reject only if a permutation test based on T also accepts or rejects.

CHAPTER 6

Categorical Data

6.1. Contingency Tables

In many experiments and in almost all surveys, many if not all of the results fall into categories rather than being measurable on a continuous or ordinal scale: e.g., male vs. female; black vs. Hispanic vs. oriental vs. white; in favor vs. against vs. undecided. The corresponding hypotheses concern proportions: "Blacks are as likely to be Democrats as they are to be Republicans." Or, "the dominant genotype 'spotted shell' occurs with three times the frequency of the recessive."

6.2. Fisher's Exact Test

As an example, suppose on examining the cancer registry in a hospital, we uncovered the following data which we put in the form of a 2 × 2 contingency table:

	Survived	Died	
Men	9	1	10
Women	4	10	14
	13	11	24

There are two rows and two columns in this table for a total of four cells. The four cell entries are 9, 1, 4, and 10. The 9 denotes the number of males who survived, the 1 denotes the number of males who died, and so forth. The four marginal totals or marginals are 10, 14, 13, and 11. The 10 is the total number of men in the study, the 14 denotes the total number of women, and so forth.

We see in this table an apparant difference in the survival rates for men and women: Only 1 of 10 men died following treatment, but 10 of the 14 women failed to survive. Is this difference statistically significant?

The answer is yes. Let's see why, using the same line of reasoning that R.A. Fisher advanced at the annual Christmas meeting of the Royal Statistical Society in 1934. (After Fisher's talk was concluded, incidentally, a seconding speaker compared his talk to "the braying of the Golden Ass." I hope you will take more kindly to my own explanation.) The preceding contingency table has several fixed elements—the total number of men in the survey, 10; the total number of women, 14; the total number who died 11, and the total number who survived 13. These totals are immutables; no swapping of labels will alter the total number of individual men and women or bring back the dead. But these totals do not determine the contents of the table as can be seen from the two tables with identical *marginal* totals that are reproduced below.

	Survived	Died	
Men	10	0	10
Women	3	11	14
	13	11	24

	Survived	Died	
Men	8	2	10
Women	5	9	14
	13	11	24

The first of these tables makes a strong case for the superior fitness of the male, stronger even than our original observations. In the second table, the survival rates for men and women are closer together than they were in our original table.

Fisher would argue that if the survival rates were the same for both sexes, then each of the redistributions of labels to subjects—that is, each of the N possible contingency tables with these same four fixed marginals—is equally likely, where

$$N = \sum_{x=0}^{10} \binom{13}{x}\binom{11}{10-x}$$
$$= \binom{13+11}{10}$$

How did we get this value for N? The component terms are taken from the hypergeometric distribution:

$$\sum_{x=0}^{t} \binom{m}{x}\binom{n}{t-x} \Big/ \binom{m+n}{t}$$ (6.1)

where n, m, t, and x occur as the indicated elements in the following 2×2 contingency table

	CAT 1	CAT 2	
CAT A	x	$t-x$	t
CAT B	$m-x$	$\cdots$	$\cdots$
	m	n	$m+n$

In our example, $m = 13$, $n = 11$, and $t = 10$, so that $S = \binom{13}{10} + 11\binom{13}{9}$ of the N tables are as or more extreme than our original table. But this is a very small fraction of the total. A difference in survival rates as extreme as the difference we observed in our original table is very unlikely to have occurred by chance. Consequently, we reject the hypothesis that the survival rates for the two sexes are the same and accept the alternative that, in this instance at least, males are more likely to profit from treatment.

I have already noted that Fisher's original presentation of this concept was marked by acrimony and dissent. You may wonder what all the fuss was about. Fisher's exact test agrees asymptotically with the chi-square test based on one degree of freedom, a fact that is no longer in dispute. But many of the participants at the meeting raged over whether there should be three or four degrees of freedom corresponding to the number of marginals or just one degree as Fisher asserted. To learn more about this controversy, see Box [X: 1978].

6.2.1. One-Tailed and Two-Tailed Tests

In the preceding example, we tested the hypothesis that survival rates do not depend on sex against the alternative that men diagnosed as having cancer are likely to live longer than women similarly diagnosed. We rejected the null hypothesis because only a small fraction of the possible tables are as extreme as the one we observed initially. This is an example of a one-tailed test. Or is it? Wouldn't we have been just as likely to reject the null hypothesis if we had observed a table of the following form:

	Survived	Died	
Men	0	10	10
Women	13	1	14
	13	11	24

Of course, we would have. In determining the significance level in the present example, we should add together the total number of tables which lie in either of the two extremes (tails) of the permutation distribution.

Recently, McKinney et al. [1989] reviewed some seventy plus articles that had appeared in six medical journals. In over half these articles, Fisher's exact test had been applied improperly. Either a one-tailed test had been used when a two-tailed test was called for or the authors of the paper simply hadn't bothered to state which test they had used.

When you design an experiment, decide at the same time whether you wish to test your hypothesis against a two-sided or a one-sided alternative. A two-sided alternative dictates a two-tailed test; a one-sided alternative dictates a one-tailed test.

As an example, suppose we decide to do a follow-on study of the cancer registry to confirm our original finding that men diagnosed as having tumors live significantly longer than women similarly diagnosed. In this follow-on study, we have a one-sided alternative. Thus, we will analyze it using a one-tailed test rather than the two-tailed test we used in the original study.

6.2.2. Increasing the Power

Providing we are willing to randomize on the boundary (see Section 2.2.3), Fisher's exact test is uniformly most powerful among all unbiased tests for comparing two binomial populations [Lehmann, 1986, pp. 151–162].

It is most powerful under any of the following four world views:

  i) binomial sampling—one set of marginals in the contingency table is random; the other set and the sum $s = n + m$ are fixed;
 ii) independent Poisson processes—all marginals and s are random;
iii) multinomial sampling—all marginals are random and s fixed;
 iv) an experiment in which sampling is replaced by the random assignment of subjects to treatments—all marginals are fixed.

The power of Fisher's test depends strongly on the composition of the sample. A balanced sample, with equal numbers in each category is the most desirable. If the sample is too unbalanced—for example, if 100 of the observations have the attribute A and only 1 has the attribute not A—it may not be possible to determine if attribute B is independent of A.

If you have some prior knowledge about the frequency of A and B, then Berkson has suggested and Neyman has proved it is better to select samples of equal size from B and not B provided $|p_B - 1/2| > |p_A - 1/2|$. The "blind faith" method of selecting the sample at random from the population at large is worse than taking equal-sized samples from either A and not A or B and not B.

Studies of the power of Fisher's exact test against various alternatives were conducted by Haber [1987], and Irony and Pereira [1986].

Although tables for determining the significance level of Fisher's exact test are available, in Finney [1948] and Latscha [1953] for example, these are restricted to a few discrete p-values. Today, it is usually much faster to compute a significance level than it is to look it up in tables. Beginning with Leslie [1955], much of the subsequent research on Fisher's exact test has been devoted to developing algorithms that would speed up or reduce the number of computations required to obtain a significance level.

As one rapid alternative to the hypergeometric distribution (equation 6.1), we may use the recursive relationship provided by Feldman and Kluger [1963]: With table entries (a_0, b_0, c_0, d_0), define

$$p_0 = \frac{(a_0 + b_0)!(a_0 + c_0)!(d_0 + b_0)!(d_0 + c_0)!}{N!a_0!b_0!c_0!d_0!}$$

it is easy to see that

$$p_{i+1} = \frac{a_i d_i}{b_{i+1} c_{i+1}} p_i$$

where $a_i = a_0 - i$.

6.2.3. The Common Odds Ratio Test

Circumstances may compel us to gather data from several test sites, for example, if we are studying the effects of treatment on a relatively rare disease. We would like to know if we are justified in combining the results from the several sites. The individual response probabilities to treatment may not be and, in fact, needn't be the same from site to site. What is essential if we are to combine the results is that the odds ratios ϕ_i

$$\frac{\pi_{iB}}{(1 - \pi_{iB})} * \frac{(1 - \pi_{iA})}{\pi_{iA}}$$

be the same, where π_{iA}, π_{iB} denote the true rates of response to treatments A and B at site i, $i = 1, \ldots, l$.

The ith site gives rise to the contingency table

$$x_i \qquad m_i - x_i$$

$$x_i' \qquad m_i - x_i'$$

To test the hypothesis $\phi_1 = \phi_2 = \cdots = \phi_l = \phi$ and, subsequently, to test that $\phi = \phi_0$, Mehta, Patel, and Gray [1985] suggest we use the permutation distribution of the statistic $T = \sum a_i(x_i)$, where

$$a_i(x_i) = -\log\left\{\binom{m_i}{x_i}\binom{m_i'}{x_i'} \middle/ \binom{m_i + m_i'}{N_i}\right\},$$

A microcomputer program to obtain confidence intervals for the common odds ratio is described by Vollset and Hirji [P: 1991].[1]

6.3. Unordered $r \times c$ Contingency Tables

6.3.1. Choosing a Test Statistic

The principal issue in the analysis of a contingency table with $r(\geq 2)$ rows and $c(\geq 2)$ columns is deciding on an appropriate test statistic. Our discussion parallels that of Agresti and Wackerly [1977]:

We can find the probabilities of any individual $r \times c$ contingency table through a straightforward generalization of the hypergeometric distribution [Halter, 1969]. An $r \times c$ contingency table consists of a set of frequencies $\{f_{ij}, 1 \leq i \leq r; 1 \leq j \leq c\}$ with row marginals $\{f_{i.}, 1 \leq i \leq r\}$ and column marginals $\{f_{.j}, 1 \leq j \leq c\}$.

$$p' = \Pr\{f'_{ij}|f_{i.}, f_{.j}\} = Q(x)/R(x) \tag{6.2}$$

with

$$Q(x) = \prod_{i=1}^{r} f_{i.}! \prod_{j=1}^{c} f_{.j}!/f_{..}!$$

and

$$R(x) = \prod_{i=1}^{r} \prod_{j=1}^{c} f_{ij}!$$

An obvious extension of Fisher's exact test is the Freeman and Halton [1951] test based on the proportion p of tables for which p' is less than or equal to the probability p_0 of the original table

$$p = \sum I(p' \leq p_0)p'$$

where the indicator $I(A) = 1$ if A is true and 0 otherwise.

While this extension may be obvious, it is not as obvious that this extension offers any protection against the alternatives of interest. Just because one table is less likely than another under the null hypothesis does not mean it is going to be more likely under the alternative. As we shall see in Section 14.1, it is the likelihood ratio P^K/P^H that is decisive. For example, consider the 1×3 contingency table $f_1 f_2 f_3$, which corresponds to the multinomial with probabilities $p_1 + p_2 + p_3 = 1$; the table whose entries are 1 2 3 argues more in favor of the null hypothesis $p_1 = p_2 = p_3$ than of the ordered alternative $p_1 > p_2 > p_3$.

---

[1] The P preceding a date, as in March, P:1972, refers to a separate bibliography at the end of the text devoted exclusively to computational methods.

The classic statistic for independence in a contingency table with r rows and c columns is

$$\chi^2 = \frac{\sum_{i=1}^{m} (v_i - Ev_i)^2}{Ev_i}.$$

Asymptotically this statistic has the chi-square distribution with $(r - 1) \cdot (c - 1)$ degrees of freedom. But for any finite sample, the chi-square distribution is only an approximation to this statistic, an approximation that is notoriously inexact for small and unevenly distributed samples. In practice, it often is necessary to combine or eliminate categories to make the chi-square approximation valid.

The permutation statistic $p_\chi = \sum I(\chi^2 \le \chi_0^2)p'$ provides an exact test and possesses all the advantages of the original chi-square. The distinction between the two approaches, as we observed in Section 2.3, is that with the original chi-square we look up the significance level in a table, while with the permutation statistic, we derive the significance level from the permutation distribution. With large samples, the two approaches are equivalent, as the permutation distribution converges to the tabulated distribution (see Chapter 14 of Bishop, Fienberg, and Holland [X: 1975]).

This permutation test has one of the original chi-square test's disadvantages: while it offers global protection against a wide variety of alternatives, it offers no particular protection against any single one of them. The statistics p and p_χ treat row and column categories symmetrically and no attempt is made to distinguish between cause and effect. To address this deficiency, Goodman and Kruskal [X: 1954] introduce an asymmetric measure of association for nominal scale variables called tau τ which measures the proportional reduction in error obtained when one variable, the "cause" or independent variable, is used to predict the other, the "effect" or dependent variable.

Assuming the independent variable determines the row,

$$\tau = \frac{\sum_j f_{mj} - f_{m\cdot}}{f_{\cdot\cdot} - f_{m\cdot}}$$

where $f_{mj} = \max_i f_{ij}$ and $f_{m\cdot} = \max_i f_{i\cdot}$.

$0 \le \tau \le 1$. $\tau = 0$ when the variables are independent: $\tau = 1$ when for each category of the independent variables all observations fall into exactly one category of the dependent. These points are illustrated in the following 2×3 tables:

3	6	9	
6	12	18	$\tau = 0$
18	0	0	
0	36	0	$\tau = 1.$
3	6	9	
12	18	6	$\tau = 0.166$

A permutation test of independence is based upon the proportion of tables for which $\tau > \tau_0$, $p_\tau = \sum I (\tau \geq \tau_0) p'$.

Cochran's Q provides an alternate test for independence. Suppose we have I experimental subjects on each of whom we administer J tests. Let $y_{ij} = 1$ or 0 denote the outcome of the jth test on the ith patient. Define

$$R_i = j y_{ij}$$

$$C_j = i y_{ij}$$

$$Q = \frac{\sum (C_j - C.)^2}{(R. - \sum (R_i)^2)}$$

Details of the calculation of the distribution of Cochran's Q under the assumption of independence are given in Patil [1975]. For a description of other, alternative statistics for use in $r \times c$ contingency tables, see Nguyen [1985].

6.3.2. Examples

We illustrate many of these points in the following two examples. The first example compares the chi-square approximation with the exact significance levels of the permutation test. The second, the categorical analysis of multivariate data, underlines the need to consult original data sources rather than summary tables.

6.3.2.1. EXACT SIGNIFICANCE LEVELS

Table 6.1 contains data on oral lesions in three regions of India derived from Gupta et al. [X: 1980] by Mehta and Patel [1990]. We want to test the hypothesis that the location of oral lesions is unrelated to geographical region. Possible test statistics include Freeman–Halton p, p_χ, and p_λ. This

Table 6.1. Oral Lesions in Three Regions of India

Site of Lesion	Kerala	Gujarat	Andhra
Labial Mucosa	0	1	0
Buccal Mucosa	8	1	8
Commissure	0	1	0
Gingiva	0	1	0
Hard Palate	0	1	0
Soft Palate	0	1	0
Tongue	0	1	0
Floor of Mouth	1	0	1
Alveolar Ridge	1	0	1

Note: Reprinted from the StatXact manual with permission from Cytel Software.

Table 6.2. Three Tests of Independence

Statistic	χ^2	$F-H$	LR
Exact *p*-value	.0269	.0101	.0356
Tabulated *p*-value	.1400	.2331	.1060

Note: Reprinted from the StatExact manual with permission from Cytel Software.

latter statistic is based on the likelihood ratio

$$\sum\sum f_{ij}\log(f_{ij}f_{..}/f_{i.}f_{.j}).$$

We may calculate the exact significance levels of these test statistics by deriving their permutation distributions or use asymptotic approximations obtained from tables of the chi-square statistic. Table 6.2 taken from Mehta and Patel [1990] compares the various approaches.

The exact significance level varies from 1% to 3.5% depending on which test statistic we select. The tabulated *p*-values vary from 11% to 23%. In one instance, the Freeman–Halton statistic, the permutation test tells us the differences among regions are significant at the 1% level; the chi-square approximation says no, they are insignificant even at the 20% level. Which answer is correct? That of the permutation test. With so many near-zero entries in the original contingency table, the chi-square approximation is not appropriate.

The results in Table 6.2 were obtained with the aid of the StatXact program for the IBM-PC. See Section 12.2 for a further description of this invaluable program.

6.3.2.2. WHAT SHOULD WE RANDOMIZE?

Table 6.3A summarizes Clarke's [X: 1960, 1962] observations on the relation between habitat and the relative frequencies of different varieties of *C. nemoralis* snail. It is tempting to analyze this table using the methods of the preceding section. But before we can analyze a data set, we need to understand *how* it was collected. In this instance, observers went to a series of locations in southern England. At each location, they noted the type of habitat—beechwoods, grasslands, and so forth, and the frequencies of each

Table 6.3A. Summary of Clarke's [X: 1960, 1962] data on C. numorialis

Habitat	N1	N2	N3	N4	N5	N6	N7	N8	N9	N10	N11	N12
Beechwoods	9	1	34	26	0	46	8	59	126	6	40	115
Other deciduous	10	1	1	0	0	85	8	13	44	2	1	12
Fens	73	3	8	4	6	89	1	23	21	11	0	22
Hedgerows	76	15	32	19	36	98	3	12	8	14	1	18
Grasslands	49	29	75	7	28	23	17	60	12	14	14	24

of twelve different varieties of snail. The original findings are summarized in Table 6.3B reproduced from Manly [1983]. Note that each row in this table corresponds to a single multivariate observation.

Manly computed the chi-square statistic for the original data as summarized in Table 6.3A. Then, using the information in Table 6.3B, he randomly reassigned the location labels to different habitats, preserving the number of locations at each habitat. For example, in one of the rearrangements, the four locations Clipper Down Wood, Boarstall Wood, Hatford, Charlbury Hill and only these four locations were designated as Fens. He formed a summary table similar to 6.3A for each rearrangement and computed the chi-square statistic for that table. He found the original value of the chi-square statistic 1757.9 was greater than any of the values he observed in each of 500 random reassignments and concluded that habitat type has a significant effect on the distribution of the various body types of the $C.$ nemoralis snail.

Manly's analysis combines multivariate and categorical techniques. It makes optimal use of all the data because it takes into account how the data was collected. Could Manly have used Table 6.3A alone to analyze the data? No, because this table lacks essential information about interdependencies among the various types of snail.

6.3.3. Underlying Assumptions

The assumptions that underlie the analysis of an $r \times c$ contingency table are the same as those that underlie the analysis of the r-sample problem. To see this, note that a contingency table is merely a way of summarizing a set of N bivariate observations. We may convert from this table to r distinct samples by using the first or row observation as the sample or treatment label and the second or column observation as the "value." Keeping the marginals fixed while we rearrange the labels ensures that the r sample sizes and the N individual values remain unchanged.

As in the r-sample problem, the labels must be exchangeable under the null hypothesis. This entails two assumptions: first, that the row and column scores are mutually independent; and second, that the observations themselves are independent of one another. We as statisticians can only test the first of these assumptions. We rely on the investigator to ensure that the latter assumption is satisfied. (See question 3 at the end of this chapter.)

6.3.4. Speeding Up the Computations

We may speed up the computations of all the preceding statistics on noting that $Q(x)$ in equation 6.2 is invariant under permutations that leave the marginals intact. Thus, we may neglect $Q(x)$ in calculating the permutation distribution and focus on $R^{-1}(x)$ [March, P: 1972].

Table 6.3B. Clarke's [1960, 1962] data* on C. nemoralis.

Habitat type	Location	N1	N2	N3	N4	N5	N6	N7	N8	N9	N10	N11	N12
Beechwoods	Clipper Down Wood	1	0	0	0	0	8	0	1	12	1	0	0
	Hackpen Wood	0	0	5	4	0	0	0	5	20	0	1	1
	Kingstone Coombes	0	0	0	2	0	4	1	0	0	0	0	2
	Danks Down Wood	0	0	2	0	0	9	0	15	21	0	1	27
	Fawley Bottom Wood	0	1	0	0	0	5	3	0	2	3	0	0
	Maidensgrove Wood	0	0	0	0	0	3	2	0	5	2	0	0
	Aston Rowant Wood	0	0	0	0	0	6	1	0	23	0	0	0
	Rockley Wood	0	0	10	15	0	0	0	4	20	0	0	21
	Manton Wood	0	0	3	1	0	0	1	6	2	0	3	9
	Knoll Down A	3	0	0	0	0	8	0	9	2	0	35	47
	Knoll Down B	0	0	7	4	0	0	0	0	0	0	0	8
	Roundway Wood	5	0	7	0	0	3	0	19	20	0	0	0
Other deciduous woods	Boarstall Wood	0	0	0	0	0	13	0	9	28	1	0	0
	Rockley Copse	9	1	1	0	0	63	8	4	10	0	0	8
	Elsfield Covert	1	0	0	0	0	6	0	0	4	0	0	0
	Uffington Wood 2	0	0	0	0	0	3	0	0	2	1	1	4
Fens	Shippon	54	1	3	3	1	54	0	8	13	7	0	20
	Headington Wick	5	1	3	0	2	14	1	13	4	2	0	0
	Cothill Fen	2	1	1	0	1	3	0	0	1	1	0	0
	Shippon Fen 2	12	0	1	1	2	18	0	2	3	1	0	2
Hedgerows and rough herbage	Hatford	1	1	0	15	0	2	0	1	3	2	0	4
	Shepherd's Rest 1	16	7	9	0	19	11	1	0	0	6	0	0
	Shepherd's Rest 2	13	4	4	0	9	0	1	0	0	1	0	0
	Standford in Vale	5	0	0	0	0	5	0	1	4	0	0	0
	Wootton	2	0	3	0	0	7	0	1	0	0	0	0

	N1	N2	N3	N4	N5	N6	N7	N8	N9	N10	N11	N12
Chisledon	6	2	0	2	4	9	0	0	0	1	0	1
Faringdon	18	0	8	0	1	34	0	5	0	0	1	4
The Ham	8	0	2	1	1	1	0	1	0	0	0	9
Wanborough Plain	2	0	0	0	0	24	1	0	1	3	0	0
Watchfield	3	1	0	0	0	2	0	0	0	1	0	0
Hill Barn Tumulus	1	0	5	0	0	0	0	3	0	0	0	0
Little Hinton	1	0	1	1	2	3	0	0	0	0	0	0
Crasslands												
Charlbury Hill	2	0	5	1	0	1	0	4	7	0	0	5
White Horse 1	4	10	4	0	3	3	3	7	0	1	2	1
White Horse 2	6	6	10	0	0	0	0	0	0	0	0	0
White Horse 3	7	2	12	0	7	7	4	5	0	2	0	0
White Horse 4	7	0	2	0	2	0	1	1	0	0	0	0
Dragons Hill 1	2	4	5	0	0	3	4	19	0	5	2	4
Dragons Hill 2	1	1	6	0	0	0	1	4	0	0	2	2
Dragons Hill 3	1	2	3	0	2	2	3	12	0	1	0	4
West Down 1	0	1	4	3	1	0	0	0	0	0	7	2
West Down 2	0	0	5	3	0	0	0	0	1	1	0	5
Sparsholt Down	13	1	15	0	6	0	0	0	0	0	0	0
Little Hinton	5	0	1	0	5	5	0	1	3	1	0	0
White Horse 5	0	2	2	0	0	1	1	1	0	0	1	0
Dragons Hill 4	1	0	2	0	2	1	1	6	1	2	0	1

* The morph types are similar to those for *hortensis*, with up to five bands present. They are: N1, yellow fully banded (Y12345); N2, yellow part-banded (N00345); N3, yellow mid-banded (Y00300); N4, yellow unbanded (Y00000); N5, other yellows; N6, pink fully banded (P12345); N7, pink part-banded (P00345); N8, pink mid-banded (P00300); N9, pink unbanded (P00000); N10, other pinks; N11, brown banded; N12, brown unbanded.

Note: From "Analysis of Polymorphic Variation in Different Types of Habitat" by BFJ Mainly, which appeared in *Biometrics*; 1983; 16: 13–27. Reprinted with permission from the Biometric Society.

We may use a recursive algorithm developed by Gail and Mantel [P: 1977] to speed up the computations for $r \times 2$ contingency tables. If $N_i(f_{\cdot 1}; f_{1 \cdot}, \ldots, f_{i \cdot})$ denotes the number of tables with the indicated marginals, then

$$N_{i+1}(f_{\cdot 1}; f_{1 \cdot}, \ldots, f_{i \cdot}, f_{i+1 \cdot}) = \sum_j N_i(f_{\cdot 1} - j; f_{1 \cdot}, \ldots, f_{i \cdot}).$$

The algorithms we developed in Chapters 3 and 4 are much too slow, since they treat each observation as an individual value.

Algorithms for speeding up the computations of the Freeman–Halton statistic in the general $r \times c$ case are given in March [P: 1972], Gail and Mantel [P: 1977], Mehta and Patel [P: 1983, 1986a, 1986b], and Pagano and Halvorsen [P: 1981]. Details of the Mehta and Patel approach are given in Section 13.4. An efficient method for generating $r \times c$ tables with given row and column totals is provided by Patefield [1981]. See also Agresti, Wackerly and Boyett [1979] and Streitberg and Rohmed [P: 1986].

The power of the Freeman–Halton statistic in the $r \times 2$ case is studied by Krewski, Brennan, and Bickis [1984].

6.4. Ordered Contingency Tables

6.4.1. Ordered $2 \times c$ Tables

In a $2 \times c$ table, test for an ordered alternative using Pitman correlation as described in Section 3.5. The test statistic is $\sum g[j] f_{1j}$ where g is any monotone increasing function.

6.4.2. Tables with More Than Two Rows and Two Columns

In an $r \times c$ contingency table conditioned on fixed marginal totals, the outcome depends only on the $(r - 1)(c - 1)$ odds ratios

$$\phi_{ij} = \frac{p_{ij} p_{i+1, j+1}}{p_{i, j+1} p_{i+1, j}}$$

where p_{ij} is the probability of an individual being classified in row i and column j.

In a 2×2 table, conditional probabilities depend on a single odds ratio and hence one- and two-tailed tests of association are easily defined. In an $r \times c$ table there are potentially two tails corresponding to *each* of the $v = (r - 1)(c - 1)$ odds ratios. Hence, an omnibus test for no association, e.g., χ^2, might have as many as 2^v tails.

Following Patefield [1982], we consider tests of the null hypothesis of no association between row and column categories $H: \phi_{ij} = 1$ for all i, j against the alternative of a positive trend $K: \phi_{ij} \geq 1$ for all i, j.

A strong positive association in any 2×2 subtable will suggest that K rather than H is true [Lehmann X: 1966].

As in the previous section, our discussion falls naturally into two parts: 1) choosing a test statistic, 2) enumerating those tables which have a test statistic greater than or equal in value to the test statistic for the original table.

6.4.3. Which Statistic?

The two principal test statistics considered by Patefield [1982] are

$$\lambda_3 = n^{-1} \sum_i \sum_j n_{ij} x_i y_j$$

for preassigned values of the row and column scores; and

$$\lambda_2 = \sup_R \left\{ n^{-1} \sum_i \sum_j n_{ij} x_i y_j \right\}$$

where the supremum is taken over all $\{x_i, y_j\}$ satisfying the conditions

$$\sum n_{i.} x_i = 0, \quad \sum n_{.j} y_j = 0, \quad \sum n_{i.} x_i^2 = n_{..}, \quad \sum n_{.j} y_j^2 = n_{..};$$

$$x_1 \leq x_2 \leq \cdots \leq x_r; \quad y_1 \leq y_2 \leq \cdots \leq y_c;$$

Patefield finds that λ_2 has higher power than λ_3 when some but not all of the ϕ_{ij} are close to unity, whereas λ_3 has higher power than λ_2 when all the ϕ_{ij} are approximately equal.

The likelihood ratio test behaves like λ_2; the Goodman and Kruskal test of association behaves like λ_3.

At first glance, it would seem that the numerous statistical methods for testing no association between a response (the rows) and K ordered categories (the columns) fall naturally into two groups: those which make use of preassigned numerical values for the scores $\{x_i, y_j\}$ and those that don't— e.g., rank tests. Graubard and Korn [1987] show this distinction is an illusion—a rank is a score and, usually, it is far from an optimal one. Midrank scores may be completely inappropriate. They advise you to assign a numerical score based on your best understanding of the relations between columns. If the choice is not apparent, they advise equally spaced scores $(1, 2, \ldots, n)$. Always examine the midranks as scores to make sure they are reasonable before using a rank test.

6.5. Covariates

The presence of a covariate adds a third dimension to a contingency table. Bross [1964] studies the effects of treatment on the survival of premature infants. His results are summarized in the following contingency table:

Table 6.4. Effect of Treatment on
Survival of the Premature

	Dead	Recovered	Total
Placebo	6	5	11
Treatment	2	12	14
	8	17	25

These results, though suggestive, are not statistically significant.

Bross notes that survival is very much a function of a third, concomitant variable—the birth weight of the child. A lower birth weight indicates greater prematurity and, hence, greater odds against a child's survival. An analysis of treatment is out of the question unless, somehow, he can correct for the effects of birth weight.

A solution we studied in earlier chapters is to set up an experiment in which we study the effects of treatment in pairs that have been matched on the basis of birth weight. But Bross' study of the premature was not an experiment; he could only observe, not control, birth weight.

Table 6.5 depicts his first nine observations, ordered by birth weight. The last two columns of this table deserve explanation. The column headed *NI* records the number of cases in which a child of lower birth weight treated with ukinase recovered when an untreated child of higher birth weight died. Such a result is to be expected under the alternative of a positive treatment effect though it would occur only occasionally by chance under the null hypothesis.

The column headed I records the number of cases in which a untreated child of lower birth weight recovered when an child of higher birth weight treated with ukinase died. Such an event or inversion would be highly unlikely under the alternative.

Table 6.5. Effect of Treatment and Birth Weight
on Survival of the Premature

Weight	Treatment	Outcome	NI TR/PL	I PL/TR
1.08	TR	D		
1.13	TR	R	3	
1.14	PL	D		
1.20	TR	R	2	
1.30	TR	R	2	
1.40	PL	D		
1.59	TR	D		
1.69	TR	R	1	
1.88	PL	D		

As his test statistic, Bross adopts $S = (Nl - l)^2/(Nl + 1)$. Note that $Nl = 8$, $l = 0$ and $S = 8$ for the original observations. Bross computes S for each of the $\binom{9}{3}$ possible rearrangements of the treatment labels—and only the labels were changed while the pairing of birth weight with outcome was preserved. None of the other rearrangements yield as large a value of S as the original observations. Bross concludes that the treatment has a statistically significant effect on survival of the premature.

6.6. Combinations of Tables

Another way to correct for the effects of a covariate is to divide the observations into blocks, so that the value of the covariate is approximately constant within each block. Under the assumption that the odds ratio is the same for each block, Mehta, Patel, and Gray [1985] provide a method for combining the results from several 2×2 contingency tables.

For a review of the literature on higher-dimensional tables see Agresti [1992].

6.7. Questions

1. **2 × 2 table.** Referring to the literature of your own discipline, see if you can find a case where a 2×2 table with at least one entry smaller than 7 gave rise to a borderline p-value using the traditional chi-square approximation. Reanalyze this table using Fisher's exact test.

   Did the original authors use a one-tailed or a two-tailed test? Was their choice appropriate?

2. **r × 2 table.** Again, refer to the literature of your own discipline for an example where the chi-square approximation was used. Do you feel the chi-square statistic was appropriate? What statistic would you have used? Reanalyze the table using the statistic you have chosen. Use all the computational shortcuts of Section 6.3.3.

3. **Independence.** If we were to question one respondent in the presence of another, would their answers be independent? If we were to make observations on several individuals in the same household, would these observations be independent? Criticize your own past work.

4. **Sample size.** According to the *Los Angeles Times*, a recent report in the *New England Journal of Medicine* states that a group of patients with a severe bacterial infection of their blood stream who received a single intravenous dose of a genetically altered antibody had a 30% death rate compared with a 49% death rate for a group of untreated patients. How large a sample size would you require using Fisher's exact test to show that such a percentage difference was statistically significant?

   Before you start your calculations, determine whether you should be using a one-tailed or a two-tailed test.

CHAPTER 7

Dependence

The title of this chapter, "dependence," reflects our continuing emphasis on the alternative rather than on the null hypothesis. As you discover anew in this chapter, the permutation test is invaluable whether you wish to focus on one or two specific hypotheses of dependence or provide protection against a broad spectrum of alternatives.

In this chapter, we consider five models of dependence and contrast the permutation approach to each with the bootstrap approach. You learn how to apply permutation tests, tracing a real-life regression problem from start to finish. And, of particular interest to economists, you learn methods for testing for first- and higher-order correlations in stationary time series.

7.1. The Models

We consider five models of dependence in order of increasing complexity.

Model 1 (Independence): For all i, the pairs $\{X_i, Y_i\}$ are independent and identically distributed with joint probability P, and P_X, P_Y are the corresponding marginal distributions. Having observed the pairs $\{X_i, Y_i;\ i = 1, \ldots, n\}$, we wish to test the hypothesis that P is the product probability $P_X * P_Y$. Model 1 is the simplest of the five models, requiring the fewest assumptions about the data; its primary interest is theoretical rather than applied.

Model 2 (Quadrant dependence): When X is positive, Y is more likely to be positive, and vice versa. This model is appropriate when we have categorical or partially ordered data.

Model 3 (Trend): $Y_i = G[X_i] + \zeta_i$ for $i = 1, \ldots, n$; where G is a monotone function of the (single) preset variable X, and the $\{\zeta_i\}$, the errors or residuals after the function G is used to predict Y, are exchangeable random variables with zero expectations. G is a monotone increasing function of X, for example, if $x_1 > x_2$ means that $G[x_1] > G[x_2]$. Having observed the pairs $\{X_i, Y_i;$

$i = 1, \ldots, n\}$, we wish to test the hypothesis that the distribution of Y is independent of X versus the alternative that Y is stochastically increasing in X. We have already encountered this model in Chapter 4, in testing for a dose response.

Model 4 (Serial correlation): $Y_i = G[X_i] + \zeta_i$ $i = 1, \ldots, n$; where G is a continuous function of the (single) preset variable X in the sense that if X_1 is "close" to X_2 then $G[X_i]$ is "close" to $G[X_2]$, and the ζ_i are independent random variables with expectation 0. Having observed the pairs $\{X_i, Y_i; i = 1, \ldots, n\}$, we wish to test the hypothesis that the distribution of Y is independent of X versus the alternative that Y depends on X through some unknown G.

Model 5 (Known model): $Y_i = G[X_i, \beta] + \zeta_i$ $i = 1, \ldots, n$ where G is a known (arbitrary) function of X a vector of preset values, β is a vector of unknown parameters, and the $\{\zeta_i\}$ are independent variables symmetrically distributed about 0. Having observed $\{X_i, Y_i; i = 1, \ldots, n\}$, we wish to test the adequacy of some estimate $\hat{\beta}$ of β, the true parameter value.

7.2. Testing for Independence

7.2.1. Independence

For Model 1, P is the product probability $P_X * P_Y$; distribution-free bootstrap and randomization tests in the spirit of Kolmogorov–Smirnov test statistics are provided by Romano [1989]. Under the assumption that the pairs $\{Y_i, X_i\}$ are independent and identically distributed, Romano finds that the bootstrap and the rerandomization test lead to almost the same confidence intervals for very large sample sizes.

Against parametric alternatives, the most powerful and/or locally most powerful tests are permutation tests based on the likelihood function [Bell and Doksum, 1967].

7.2.2. Quadrant Dependence

In Model 2, no ordinal relationship is implied; X and Y may even take categorical values, so that the problem reduces to that of analyzing a 2×2 contingency table. The most powerful permutation test and, not incidentally, the most powerful unbiased test is Fisher's exact test described in Section 6.2.

The bootstrap for the 2×2 contingency table may be determined entirely on theoretical grounds without the need to resort to resampling. Estimates of the probabilities $P\{Y > 0 | X > 0\}$, and $P\{Y > 0 | X < 0\}$ are used to obtain a confidence interval for the odds ratio. If this interval contains unity, we accept the null hypothesis of independence, otherwise we reject it in favor of the alternative of quadrant dependence.

This model is occasionally used in practice while exploring the relationship between X and Y, first transforming to the deviations about the sample mean, $X_i' = X_i - \overline{X}$, $Y_i' = Y_i - \overline{Y}$.

7.3. Testing for Trend

Consider an experiment in which you make two disparate observations on each of a series of experimental subjects. For example, observing the birth weight of an infant and its weight after one year; or the blood pressure and caffeine intake of each of a series of adults. You wish to test the hypothesis that the two variables vary independently against the alternative that there is a positive dependence between them.

More accurately, you wish to test the alternative of positive dependence against the null hypothesis of independence. In formal terms, if X and Y are the two variables, and Y_x is the random variable whose distribution is the conditional distribution of Y given that $X = x$, we want to test the null hypothesis that Y_x has the same distribution for all x, against the alternative that if $x' > x$, then $Y_{x'}$, is likely to be larger than Y_x.

In Section 14.2, we show that Pitman's correlation $\sum x_{(i)} y_i$, where $x_{(1)} \leq x_{(2)} \leq \cdots x_{(n)}$, provides a most powerful unbiased test against alternatives with a bivariate normal density. As the sample size increases, the cutoff point for Pitman's test coincides with the cutoff point for the corresponding α normal test based on the Pearson correlation coefficient.

Let's apply this test to the weight and cholesterol levels taken from a subset of the blood chemistry data collected by Werner et al. [X: 1970]; the full data set is included with the BMDP statistical package.

Wt	Chol
144	200
160	600
128	243
150	50
178	227
140	220
158	305
170	220

Is there a trend in cholesterol level by weight? Reordering the data by weight provides a clearer picture.

Wt	Chol
128	243
140	220
144	200
150	50
158	305
160	600
170	220
178	227

The cholesterol level does not appear to be related to weight; or, at least, it is not directly related. Again, we can confirm our intuition by the permutation test based on the statistic r.

But before we perform the test, what should we do about the subjects who had cholesterol values of 50 and 600? Are these typographical errors or a misreading of the test results? Should we discard these values completely or perhaps replace them by ranks? Chapter 9 is devoted to a discussion of these and other alternatives for dealing with suspect data. In this chapter, we play the data as it lays. For the original data, $r = 128 * 243 + \cdots + 178 * 227 = 320,200$, while $r = 332,476$ for the following worst-case permutation:

Wt	Chol
128	50
140	200
144	220
150	220
158	227
160	243
170	305
178	600

Examining several more rearrangements, we easily confirm our eyeball intuition that cholesterol level is not directly related to weight. The majority of permutations of the data have sample correlations larger and more extreme than that of our original sample. We accept the null hypothesis.

7.4. Serial Correlation

For Model 4, advocates of the permutation test can take advantage of the (possible) local association between Y and X, reordering the X_i so that $X_1 \leq \cdots \leq X_n$, and adopting as test statistic $M = \sum_{i=i}^{n-1} (Y_i - Y_{i+1})^2$ [Wald and

Wolfowitz, 1943; Noether, 1950; Maritz, 1981, p. 219]. We reject the null hypothesis if the value of the statistic M for the original observations is less than the αth percentile of the permutation distribution of M. Again, we need not make specific assumptions about the nature of the association. If we can make specific assumptions, then some other permutation test may recommend itself. Ghosh [1954], for example, considers tests against the alternative of periodic fluctuations. Manly [1991] also considers a number of practical examples.

It is not clear what statistic, beyond that proposed by Romano for the simpler Model 1, might be used as the basis of a bootstrap test of Model 4. Of course, if we are prepared to specify the dependence function G explicitly, as is the case in Model 5, we may apply bootstrap methods to the residuals or to a suitable transformation thereof; see, for example, Stine [X: 32].

7.4.1. An Example

To see a second illustration of the regression method (Model 3) while making a novel application of the present model, let us consider a second example, this time employing hypothetical data.

In Table 7.1, X represents the independent variable or cause, and Y represents the dependent variable or effect. Plotting Y versus X as in Figure 7.1 suggests a linear trend, and our permutation test for Model 3 confirms its presence. Our next step is to formulate a specific model and to estimate its parameters. The simplest model is a linear one $Y = a + bX + \varepsilon$. We can estimate the coefficents a and b using the method of least squares.

$$b = \frac{S_{xy}}{S_{xx}} = 4.5$$

$$a = \bar{y} - b\bar{x} = 3.53,$$

where

Table 7.1. Exploring a Cause-Effect Relationship

X	Y	$a+bX$	residual	rank	$a+bX+cX^2$	residual
1	10.56	8.74	1.81	7	11.68	−1.12
2	15.28	14.15	1.12	6	14.57	.70
3	20.13	19.56	.56	5	18.31	1.82
4	22.26	24.98	−2.72	1	22.88	−0.62
5	28.06	30.38	−2.32	2	28.29	−0.23
6	33.61	35.80	−2.18	3	34.53	−0.93
7	41.13	41.20	−0.08	4	41.62	−0.49
8	50.41	46.62	3.79	8	49.55	0.86

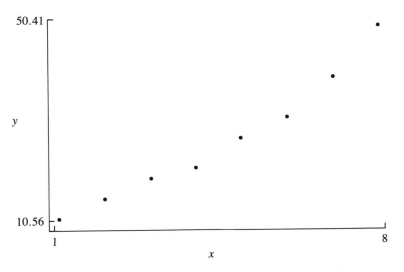

Figure 7.1. Plotting the effect Y against values of the cause X.

$$S_{xy} = \sum (x_i - \bar{x})(y_i - \bar{y})$$
$$S_{xx} = \sum (x_i - \bar{x})^2.$$

But a simple model is not always the right model. Suppose we compare our predictions from the linear model with the actual observations as in the second and third columns of our table. The fourth and final column of this table which lists the differences between the predicted and observed values attracts our interest. Is there some kind of trend here also? Examining a plot of the residuals in Figure 7.2, there does appear to be some sort of relationship between the residuals and our variable X. We can confirm the existence of this relationship by testing for serial correlation among the residuals. As a preliminary aid to the intuition, examine the ranks of the residuals in the fifth column of the table: 7 6 5 1 2 3 4 8. How likely is such a highly organized sequence to occur by chance? The value of M for the original residuals is 39.45; not one of 400 random rearrangements yields a value of M this extreme. The permutation test confirms the presence of a residual relationship not accounted for by our initial first-order model.

Let's try a second order model: $Y = a + bX + cX^2 + \varepsilon$; the least squares coefficients are $Y = 9.6 + 1.6X + 0.42X^2$; we've plotted the results in the final columns of Table 7.1; note the dramatic reduction in the size of the residuals; the second-order model provides a satisfactory fit to our data.

We could obtain bootstrap estimates of the joint distribution of X, Y by selecting random pairs, but with far less efficiency. If we are willing and justified in making additional assumptions about the nature of the trend function and the residuals as in Model 5, then a number of more powerful bootstrap tests may be formulated. While we remain in an exploratory phase,

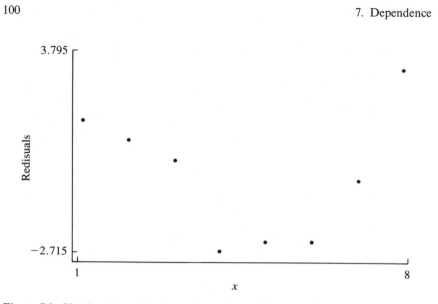

Figure 7.2. Plotting the residuals against values of the cause X after estimating and subtracting the linear trend.

our best choice of a test procedure appears to be Pitman's test followed by the Wald and Wolfowitz test for serial correlation among the residuals.

7.4.2. Trend

We can test for a trend over time by using the Pitman correlation $\sum t X(t)$, where $X(t)$ is the value of X at time t [Wald and Wolfowitz, 1943]. In the presence of a trend, the value of the test statistic should be more extreme than $1 - \alpha$ of the values $\sum \pi(t) X(t)$ where π is a permutation of the index set $\{t_1, \ldots, t_n\}$.

We reach the same decision—accept or reject—whether we use the original values of the index set, for example, the dates 1985, 1986, 1987 ... to compute our test statistic or rezero them first as in 0, 1, 2, ... For $\sum (t - C) X(t) = \sum t X(t) - C \sum X(t)$, and the latter sum is invariant under permutations of the index set.

7.4.3. First-Order Dependence

In a large number of economic and physical applications, we are willing to accept the existence of a first-order dependence in time (or space) of the form $X(t + \tau) = f[\tau] X(t) + e_{t+\tau}$ but we would like to be sure that second- and higher-order interactions are zero or close to zero. That is, if we are trying to predict $X(t)$ and already know $X(t - 1)$, we would like to be sure that no further information is to be gained from a knowledge of $X(t-2)$, $X(t-3)$, and so forth.

Gabriel [X: 1962] generalizes the issue as follows: Define $\{x(i)\}$ to be sth-degree antedependent if the partial correlation of $x(i)$ and $x(i-s-z-1),\ldots,$ $x(1)$ for $x(i-1),\ldots,x(i-s-z)$ held constant is zero for all nonnegative z.

To test the hypothesis H_s that the $\{x(i)\}$ are sth antedependent against the alternative H_{s+1}, accept H_s if

$$R = -N \sum_{i=1}^{p-s-1} \ln(1 - r^2_{i,i+1,\ldots,i+s})$$

is small. We can assess R against its permutation distribution over time or, if we have $25+$ observations, follow Gabriel [X: 1962] and make use of a chi-square approximation.

7.5. Known Models

In Model 5, we may be given the vector of parameters β or we may need to estimate it. We consider the testing problem first. Confidence intervals for the parameters are covered in Section 7.5.2.

7.5.1. Testing

Under the assumption of independent (but perhaps not identically distributed) symmetrically distributed residuals, we may form an unbiased permutation test of the hypothesis $F = G_\beta$ by permuting the signs of the deviations $d_i = Y_i - G_{\hat{\beta}}(X_i)$ to obtain the distribution of the statistic

$$M = \sum_+ L[d_{\pi(i)}],$$

where $\sum_+$ ranges over the set for which $d_{\pi(i)} \geq 0$. A confidence interval for the unknown β can be obtained using the method described in Section 7.3.

At least three bootstrap procedures compete for our attention: First, we may resample from the residuals as we do in the case of censored matched pairs (see Section 9.4) and test the hypothesis that the mean (or the median) of the residuals is zero. The resultant test is inferior to the permutation test; it is markedly inferior if the residuals have markedly different variances.

Second, we may resample from the $\{Y_i, X_i\}$ and obtain a series of bootstrap estimates β^*; in this case, the d_i need not be identically distributed. Or, third, for each X_i, we may resample from the d_i to obtain a Y_i', and use the $\{Y_i', X_i\}$ to estimate β; providing, that is, we can assume that the d_i are identically distributed. By resampling repeatedly, using one or the other of these latter two methods, we may obtain a confidence region for β and thus a test for our original hypothesis.

Three points require additional clarification:

1) The method of estimation.
2) The confidence region. In some applications, for example, when the $\{X_i\}$ are almost colinear, a "figure 8" may be more natural than an ellipsoid. Can this region be optimized "against" specific alternatives?
3) The weighting to be given the various parameters. For large samples, a normal approximation suggests the use of a covariance matrix for weighting purposes. For small samples, the issue may not be resolvable.

As a result of these unresolved issues, bootstrap confidence intervals and the associated tests of hypotheses for the generalized regression problem are still a matter of considerable controversy.

For Model 5, the permutation test and the bootstrap may lead to quite different results. While the boostrap can take advantage of the parametric structure of a problem, (if one is known), the permutation test spares us the necessity for making decisions about parameters concerning which we have little or no information.

7.5.2. Confidence Intervals

In most cases, it is not enough to know that Y is dependent on X, we want to know the specific nature of this dependence. As an example, suppose we have satisfied ourselves that Model 3 (Trend) holds—that is $Y_i = G[X_i] + \zeta_i$ for $i = 1, \ldots, n$, where G is a monotone function of the (single) preset variable X, $G = a + bX$, say and the ζ_i are exchangeable random variables with zero expectations. Having decided that $b \neq 0$, we would like to obtain a confidence interval for b. First note that a permutation test of the hypothesis $H_0: b = b_0$ may be based on the Pitman correlation

$$\sum x_i \zeta_i^0$$

where $\zeta_i^0 = y_i - y. - x_i b_0$, $i = 1, \ldots, n$ are the deviations about the line whose slope is b_0.

Let π denote a permutation of the subscripts $1, \ldots, n$ and put $b^\pi[w] = \sum x_i w_{\pi[i]} / \sum \xi_i^2$. For example,

$$b^\pi[\zeta^0] = \sum x_i \zeta_{\pi[i]}^0 / \sum \xi_i^2$$

We reject or accept H_0 according to whether $b^I[\zeta^0]$ for the original, unpermuted deviations is or is not an extreme value of the distribution of $b^\pi[\zeta^0]$.

We can obtain a confidence interval for b by following the trial and error procedure described in Section 3.2. But there is a better way, due to Robinson [1987]:

The least squares estimate of b is $\hat{b} = \sum x_i y_i / \sum \xi_i^2$, so that $b^I[\zeta^0] = \hat{b} - b_0$ for the original, unpermuted deviations. Let $\hat{\zeta}_i = y_i - y. - x_i \hat{b}$;

$$\zeta_i^0 = \hat{\zeta}_i + (\hat{b} - b_0)x_i;$$

$$b^\pi[\zeta^0] = b^\pi[\hat{\zeta}] + (\hat{b} - b_0)b^\pi[x];$$

$$\{b_0: b^\pi[\zeta^0] \geq \hat{b} - b_0\} = \{b_0: b^\pi[\hat{\zeta}] \geq (\hat{b} - b_0)(1 - b^\pi[x])\}$$

$$= \{b_0: b^\pi[\hat{\zeta}]/(1 - b^\pi[x]) \geq \hat{b} - b_0\}.$$

$b^\pi[\hat{\zeta}]/(1 - b^\pi[x])$ is a pivotal quantity that does not depend on b_0. The desired confidence region is the interval between the kth and the $(n! - k + 1)$th order statistics of this pivotal quantity where $k = (n!\alpha/2)$.

7.6. Questions

1. a) Are the bootstrap and permutation tests against quadrant dependence equivalent for very large samples?
   b) Suppose you observed the contingency table

	Republican	Democrat
White	8	3
Black	3	8

   Is race associated with political preference? Use both the bootstrap and Fisher's Exact test (Section 6.2) to make the inference.

2. In your own area of specialization, there is undoubtedly a controversy about the nature of the association between some pair of variables. Which of the models, 1? 2?, ..., 5? would be most appropriate for describing this association?

3. Adding platinum to a metallic coating will increase the mean time between failures. But is it worth it? This will depend on the cost of platinum, the magnitude of the effect, and the cost of a failure. Using the data in the following table and the prediction equation MTBF $= a + b(PT)$, obtain a confidence interval for the effect b. Use both the trial and error method (Section 3.2) and the pivotal quantity developed in Section 7.4.

Table 7.2. Effect of Platinum on MTBF

Grams Platinum per KG	MTBF (Hours)
1	900
2	1000
5	1100
10	1300
15	1600
20	1800

4. a) Table 7.3 records monthly sales for a two year period, taken from Makridakis, Wheelwright, and McGee [1983]. Is there a seasonal trend?

Table 7.3. Monthly Sales as a Function of X

t	X	Sales	t	X	Sales
0	116.44	202.66	12	129.85	260.51
1	119.58	232.91	13	122.65	266.34
2	125.74	272.07	14	121.64	281.24
3	124.55	290.97	15	127.24	286.19
4	122.35	299.09	16	132.35	271.97
5	120.44	296.95	17	130.86	265.01
6	123.24	279.49	18	122.90	274.44
7	127.99	255.75	19	117.15	291.81
8	121.19	242.78	20	109.47	290.91
9	118.00	255.34	21	114.34	264.95
10	121.81	271.58	22	123.72	228.40
11	126.54	268.27	23	130.33	209.33

b) After eliminating the seasonal trend from the sales data in Table 1, is there a significant upward trend in the remaining averages? Your test statistic is what sum?

c) The "X" of Table 1 is actually advertising expenditures. Can a knowledge of your advertising expenditures explain part of the trend in sales? What statistic would you use to determine if sales do depend on advertising X.

d) Should you test this multivariate regression before eliminating the seasonal trend? Would the sales in month i depend on the advertising expenditures in month i? or the previous month $i - 1$? Or on those in several previous months? What statistics would you use to resolve these issues?

CHAPTER 8

Clustering in Time and Space

In this chapter, you learn how to detect clustering in time and space and to validate clustering models. We use the generalized quadratic form in its several guises including Mantel's U and Mielke's multi-response permutation procedure to work through a series of applications in atmospheric science, epidemiology, ecology, and archeology.

8.1. The Generalized Quadratic Form

8.1.1. Mantel's U

Mantel's U [Mantel, 1967] $\sum \sum a_{ij}b_{ij}$ is perhaps the most widely used of all multivariate statistics. In Mantel's original formulation, a_{ij} is a measure of the temporal distance between items i and j, while b_{ij} is a measure of the spatial distance. As an example, suppose the pair (t_i, l_i) represents the day t_i on which the ith individual in a study came down with cholera and $l_i = (l_{i1}, l_{i2})$ denotes her position in space. For all i, j set $a_{ij} = 1/(t_i - t_j)$ and

$$b_{ij} = 1/\sqrt{(l_{i1} - l_{j1})^2 + (l_{i2} - l_{j2})^2}$$

A large value for U would support the view that cholera spreads by contagion from one household to the next. How large is large? As always, we compare the value of U for the original data with the values obtained when we fix the i's but permute the j's as in $U' = \sum \sum a_{ij}b_{i\pi(j)}$.

The generalized quadratic form has seen widespread application in anthropology, archaeology [Klauber, 1971, 1975], ecology [Bryant, 1977; Douglas and Endler, 1982; Highton, 1977; Levin, 1977; Royaltey, Astrachen, and Sokal, 1975; Ryman et al., 1980], education [Schultz and Hubert, 1976], epidemiology [Alderson and Nayak, 1971; Fraumeni and Li, 1969; Glass and Mantel, 1969; Klauber and Mustacchi 1970; Kryscio et al., 1973; Mantel and

Bailar, 1970; Merrington and Spicer, 1969; Siemiatycki and McDonald, 1972; Smith and Pike, 1976; Till et al., 1967], geography [Cliff and Ord, 1971, 1973, 1981; Hubert, 1978b; Hubert, Golledge, and Costanzo, 1981; Hubert et al., 1984, 1985], management science [Graves and Whinston, 1970], psychology [Hubert and Schultz 1976; Hubert, 1978a, 1979], sociology [Hubert and Baker, 1978], and systematics [Dietz, 1983; Gabriel and Sokal, 1969; Jones, Selander, and Schnell, 1980; Selander and Kaufman, 1975; Sokal, 1979].

8.1.2. An Example

An ongoing fear among many parents is that something in their environment —asbestos or radon in the walls of their house, or toxic chemicals in their air and ground water, will affect their offspring. Table 8.1 is extracted from data collected by Siemiatycki and McDonald [1972] on congenital neural-tube defects. Eyeballing the gradient along the diagonal of this table one might infer that ancephalic births occur in clusters. One could test this hypothesis statistically using the methods of Chapter 6 for ordered categories, but a better approach, since the exact time and location of each event is known, is to use Mantel's U. The question arises as to which measures of distance and time we should employ. Mantel [1967] reports striking differences between one analysis of epidemiologic data in which the coefficients are proportional to the differences in position and a second approach (which he recommends) to the same data in which the coefficients are proportional to the reciprocals of these differences.[1] Using Mantel's approach, a pair of infants born 5 kilometers and 3 months apart contribute $\frac{1}{3} * \frac{1}{5} = 1/15$ to the correlation. Summing up the contributions from all pairs, then repeating the summing process for a series of random rearrangements, Siemiatycki and McDonald conclude that the clustering of ancephalic infants is not statistically significant.

Table 8.1. Incidents of pairs of ancephalic infants by distance and time months apart

km apart	< 1	< 2	< 4
< 1	39	101	235
< 5	53	156	364
< 25	211	652	1516

[1] One further caveat: Mantel's U fails completely if the spatial distribution of the underlying population is also changing with time [Roberson and Fisher, 1986].

8.2. Applications

By appropriately restricting the values of a_{ij} and b_{ij}, the definition of Mantel's U can be seen to include several of the standard measures of correlation including those usually attributed to Pearson, Pitman, Kendall, and Spearman [Hubert, 1985]. Mantel's U has been rediscovered frequently, often without proper attribution; see Whaley [1983]. In this section we consider three diverse approaches to the problem of assessing the presence of clustering in space and time. In each case, the permutation distribution of the quadratic form is used to provide a baseline against which the behavior of the observations may be assessed.

8.2.1. The MRPP Statistic

One such variant is the MRPP or multi-response permutation procedure [Mielke, 1979] which is used in applications as diverse as the weather and the spatial distribution of archaeological artifacts. The MRPP uses the permutation-distribution of between-object distances to determine whether a classification structure has a nonrandom distribution in space or time. With large samples, a Pearson type III curve based on the first three (or four) exact moments may be used in place of the permutation distribution [Mielke, Berry, and Brier, 1981].

An example of the application of the MRPP arises in the assignment of antiquities (artifacts) to specific classes based on their spatial locations in an archaeological dig. Presumably, the kitchen tools of primitive man—woks and Cuisinarts—should be found together, just as a future archaeologist can expect to find TV, VCR, and stereo side by side in a neolithic living room.

Following Berry et al. [1980, 1983], let $\Omega = \{\omega_1, \ldots, \omega_N\}$ designate a collection of N artifacts within a site; let $X_{1i}, \ldots, X_{ri}$ denote the r coordinates for the site space for artifact ω_i; let $S_1, \ldots, S_{g+1}$ represent an exhaustive partitioning of the N artifacts into $g + 1$ disjoint classes, (the $g + 1$st being reserved for not-yet-classified items); and let n_j be the number of artifacts in the jth class.

Define the Euclidian distance between two artifacts,

$$\delta_{ij} = \left[\sum_{k=1}^{r} (X_{ki} - X_{kj})^2 \right]^{1/2}$$

Define the average between-artifact distance for all artifacts within the ith class,

$$\zeta_i = \frac{2}{n_i(n_i - 1)} \sum_{i < j} \delta_{ij} \phi_i(\omega_i) \phi_i(\omega_j),$$

where $\phi_i(\omega)$ is an indicator function that is 1 if $\omega \in S_i$ and 0 otherwise.

The test statistic is the weighted within-class average of these distances,

$$\Delta = \sum_{i=1}^{g} n_i \zeta_i / K$$

where $K = \sum_{i=1}^{g} n_i$

The permutation distribution associated with Δ is taken over all $\dfrac{N!}{\prod_{i=1}^{g+1} n_i!}$

allocations of the N artifacts to the $g + 1$ classes with the same numbers $\{n_i\}$ assigned to each class.

Empirical power comparisons between MRPP rank tests and with other rank tests are made by Tracy and Tajuddin [1985] and Tracy and Khan [1990].

8.2.2. BW Statistic of Cliff and Ord, (1973)

As a second application of generalized correlation, suppose we want to measure the degree to which the presence of some factor in an area (or time period) increases the chances that this factor will be found in an nearby area.

The BW statistic of Cliff and Ord [1973] is defined as $\sum\sum \delta_{ij}(x_i - x_j)^2$ where

$$x_i \quad \begin{array}{l} = 1 \text{ if the } i\text{th area has the characteristic} \\ = 0 \text{ otherwise} \end{array}$$

$$\delta_{ij} \quad \begin{array}{l} = 1 \text{ if the } i\text{th and } j\text{th areas are adjacent} \\ = 0 \text{ otherwise.} \end{array}$$

8.2.3. Equivalances

The generalized quadratic form has been rediscovered and redefined in many different guises. Whaley [1983] shows that Mantel's U and the BW statistic are equivalent to the MRPP for testing purposes. A third equivalent example is the k-dimensional runs test of Friedman and Rafsky [1983] studied in Section 5.2.

8.3. Extensions

Mantei's U is quite general in its application. The sets of coefficients $\{a_{ij}\}$ and $\{b_{ij}\}$ need not represent positions or changes in time and space.

In a completely disparate application in sociology, Hubert and Schultz,

[1976], observers studied k distinct variables in each of a large number of subjects. Their object was to test a specific sociological model for the relationships among the variables. This time, the $\{a_{ij}\}$ in Mantel's U are elements of the $k \times k$ sample correlation matrix while the $\{b_{ij}\}$ are elements of an idealized or theoretical correlation matrix derived from the model. A large value of U supports the model, a small value rules against it.

8.3.1. Another Dimension

Vecchia and Iyer [1989] generalized the MRPP for use in the comparison of several linear models. In the words of these authors, "Regarding algebraic quantities useful to detect concentrations of points within distinct groups, one might have asked: *when are two points concurrent?*. The answer, that they coincide whenever the *distance between them is zero* motivates the definition of the MRPP statistic in terms of interpoint distance.

"Extending this approach, for example, to the *comparison of straight line relations*, the analogous geometric argument is that three points are colinear only if their triangular *area is zero*."

The statistic used in Vecchia and Iyer's new test is a symmetric volume: a real-valued function, symmetric in its $n + 1$ arguments, that is zero if and only if the Euclidean volume of the simplex formed by the arguments is zero. An immediate application for this statistic is assessing the consistency of multiclinic designs. Some of this statistic's asymptotic properties are considered in Vecchia and Iyer [1991].

8.4. Questions

1. Show that Pitman's correlation is a special case of Mantel's U.

2. List at least two applications for Vecchia and Iyer's test.

CHAPTER 9

Coping with Disaster

In this chapter, you receive practical guidelines for coping with the many catastrophes that confront the applied statistician:

* subjects who miss an appointment,
* subjects who disappear completely and mysteriously in the middle of an experiment,
* incomplete questionnaires,
* covariates after the fact,
* outlying observations whose extreme and questionable values suggest they may have been recorded incorrectly,
* off-scale and other censored values that can not be determined with precision,
* and even studies that must be brought to a rapid and untimely conclusion well in advance of the scheduled date.

9.1. Missing Data

The effects of missing data depend upon the nature of the study. In some instances, for example, in the one-factor, k-sample comparison, missing data has no effect upon the analysis other than to reduce the power of the test. In other, more complex designs, missing data may result in an unbalanced design in which several factors are confounded with one another. In most, though not all, of these latter cases, no special statistical procedures are required, *providing* we are careful in how we interpret the results. We must identify which effects are confounded with one another, a main effect with an interaction, say. In other studies (and one such example was examined in Section 4.4.2,) we may have to abandon permutation procedures altogether and consider using the bootstrap.

The majority of experimental designs belong to the correctable category.

We proceed with the permutation analysis using a revised set of marginal constraints that reflect the actual rather than the hoped-for sample sizes. And in analyzing the results, we acknowledge that one or more higher-order interactions may have contaminated the observed effects.

Consider an example we studied in Section 4.2, the effect of sunlight and fertilizer on crop yield. Suppose that one of the observations in the low-sunlight, medium-fertilizer group, the 22 noted in parenthesis in the table below, is missing from the study.

Effect of Sunlight and Fertilizer
on Crop Yield

	Fertilizer		
	LO	MED	HIGH
LO	5	15	21
	10	(22)	29
	8	18	25
HI	6	25	55
	9	32	60
	12	40	48

The test statistic for the main effect of sunlight $S = 23 + (15 + 8) + 75 = 131$ for these observations. Such an extremely low value is found in only a small handful of the rearrangements in which we swap observations at random between the low and high groups. The number of rearrangements after correcting for the missing data item is $\binom{17}{8}$. The reduction from the hoped for $\binom{18}{9}$ rearrangements reduced the power of the test. But the reduction is irrelevant in this instance as we are rejecting the hypothesis. Had we accepted the null hypothesis, we would have been forced to consider whether a larger sample size might have enabled us to detect an effect.

A missing data item in only one of the groups means that the main effect of sunlight is partially confounded with the interaction between sunlight and fertilizer. But our common sense strengthened by a glance at the table tells us that the confounding also is irrelevant in this instance.

The preceding discussion was based on the implicit assumption that dropouts occur at random. If the dropout rate is directly related to the treatment, we must either abandon the study or modify our scoring system explicitly to account for the dropout. See, for example, Entsuah [1990].

A further example of using the permutation distribution to cope with missing data is given in Section 10.2.6.

9.2. Covariates After the Fact

After World War II, public policy makers in the United States did a slow about-face on the dangers of tobacco smoke. The changes in policy accelerated during the 1970's. One moment it seemed the cigarette was the ultimate symbol of masculinity and the next it was the primary cause of emphysema, hypertension, lung cancer, and fetal defects. One month you could design a 400-patient, six-week, 50-variable clinical study with the full support of a Food and Drug Administration panel, and the next the panel would be asking if you'd corrected for the smokers in the control group. Of course you hadn't, not then, not in those days.

Today, we know that smoking is harmful, but "cigarettes smoked per week" is only one of hundreds of possible covariates. Regardless of how many covariates you have controlled or matched in putting together a clinical study, there are sure to be one or two more covariates that you didn't think of, that no one thought of, that no one could have envisioned—that is, until the day after your 300-page report on the study was sent to the printers.

All is not lost, it is still possible to make a comparison among treatment groups using the method of permutations by restricting the rerandomizations to those with specific after-the-fact design matrices.

Using the method due to Rosenbaum [1984], described at length in Section 4.3, we block the data into smokers and nonsmokers (or lemon eaters and non-lemon-eaters), and then randomize separately within each block.

Restricting the number of randomizations may reduce the power of the test. (It may also increase it by eliminating a source of variability; see Section 3.6.) As a result, we may need to add more subjects and an additional clinical center to the study to justify and confirm any negative results.

9.2.1. Observational Studies

An extreme example of the use of an after-the-fact covariate comes when we attempt to create matched pairs from two groups that were part of an observational study. In an observational study, the groupings themselves are after the fact. The subjects are not randomly assigned to treatment or control but are merely "observed" to belong to one group or the other. Through the use of after-the-fact covariates, we hope to reduce or eliminate any built-in biases.

An example provided by Rosenbaum [1988] is that of a study in humans of the effect of vasectomy on the risk of myocardial infarction. Obviously, we do not have the luxury (nor the authority, thankfully) to select a random sample of patients for a mandatory vasectomy, but must analyze the data as it lies. We can take advantage of concurrent data on obesity and smoking history (both of which are known to affect the risk of myocardial infarction) to help us block the two samples so as to reduce the between-sample variance. See Rosenbaum [1988] for methods for dealing with imperfect matching.

While no justification for the use of restricted randomization is required when the covariates are built in to the experimental design, formal justification for the use of Rosenbaum's method after the fact requires us to make three assumptions:

First, for all observations, the observed treatment assignment z ($z = j$ if the unit is assigned to treatment j) and the vector $r = (r_1, \ldots, r_J)$ of potential responses to treatment of that unit are conditionally independent given the vector of observed covariates. Second, regardless of the values taken by the covariates, all treatment assignments are possible. And third, the conditional probability $e[X]$ of receiving a particular treatment given a vector of observed covariates X, follows a logistic model [Cox and Shell, 1989], that is

$$\log\left\{\frac{e[X]}{(1 - e[X])}\right\} = \beta^T f(X),$$

where $f(X)$ is a known but arbitrary vector-valued function of X. Since $f(X)$ is arbitrary, this latter condition is not particularly restrictive.

All three of these assumptions are satisfied if the covariates did not affect the treatment assignment. For example, obesity and smoking history would satisfy these conditions if they were not factors in the patient/physician decision to have or perform a specific treatment.

9.3. Outliers

Consider the set of observations 0, 1, 2, 3, 19. Does the 19 represent a genuine response to treatment, the response we have been looking for, or is it an outlier—a typographical error or a bad reading that will only lead us astray? In the first case, we will want to utilize the data just as it is; in the second, we will want to modify or perhaps even to discard the questionable reading.

Shall we deal with such outliers on a one-by-one basis? Or should we establish a policy that will automatically adjust for and diminish the effect of outliers? Ad hoc rejection of suspect data could lead to charges of bias. A systematic policy can be adjusted for sample size and power determinations.

We consider six policies here:

1) preserving the original data
2) Using ranks in place of the original observations, thus diminishing the effects of outliers
3) Replacing the observations/ranks by scores derived from some standard distribution, e.g., the order statistics of a standardized normal distribution
4) applying a robust tail-compression transformation to all the data

5) censoring extreme observations
6) deleting extreme observations.

Whichever policy we elect, the permutation method will be more robust to outliers than a test based on a parametric distribution. The influence functions of a two-sample permutation test are always bounded above, even if the influence functions of the corresponding parametric test are unbounded from above and below [Lambert, 1981]. Our only concern need be the selection of a test statistic that is both practical and optimal.

9.3.1. Original Data

"The Method of Randomization applied to the original observations produced stunningly efficient tests which were dismally impractical." [Bradley, 1968]

Despite these discouraging words from James V. Bradley, I almost always make use of the original observations rather than their transform.

The exception that proves the rule is in my analysis of the Renis data considered in problem 2 of Chapter 3 and in Good [1979]. In that study, I used a preliminary logarithmic transformation, but it was to equalize the variances in the two samples, not to eliminate large values.

The computational difficulties to which Bradley alluded have largely been resolved through advances in computer technology between 1968 and today; the efficiency of the permutation test remains. The power and high relative efficiency of the permutation test comes from its use of exact values. Throw away one of the observations or replace it with its rank or a trimmed value and you reduce the power of the corresponding test. The gain in power is particularly evident when there is a mixture of responders and nonresponders [Good, 1979]; but see Boos and Browne [1986].

On the other hand, a single extreme observation often can have a disproportionate effect. Given the observations 0, 1, 2, 3, 19, would you rather guesstimate the population mean as 2 or 2.5 than estimate it using the sample mean of 5? By taking ranks or applying some other tail-compressing transformation to all the observations, we can "democratize" the data so that each data item has a relatively equal influence upon the final calculation. (See also Hampel et al. [X: 1986]).

9.3.2. Ranks

Suppose we have two samples: the first control sample takes values 0, 1, 2, 3, 15. The second treatment sample takes values 3.1, 3.5., 4., 5, and 6. Does the second sample include larger values than the first?

When we rank the data giving the smallest observation a rank of 1, the next smallest the rank of 2, and so forth, the first sample includes the ranks 1,

2, 3, 4, 10 and the second sample includes the ranks 5, 6, 7, 8, 9. Does the second sample include larger values than the first?

Applying the two-sample comparison described in Chapter 3.2 to the ranked data, we conclude at the 10% level that the second sample is significantly larger. The sums of the ranks in the original first sample, 20, is as large or larger in just 24 of the $\binom{10}{5} = 252$ rearrangements.

Obviously, taking ranks diminishes the effects of outliers. Taking ranks has a second advantage from the computational point of view: When we take ranks, the results are unconditionally distribution free. As we are working with the same values—the ranks, over and over regardless of the actual values of the observations, we can tabulate the significance levels of our test statistics (at least for small samples) and avoid lengthy computations. And we may determine analytically when a sample of ranks is large enough that its permutation distribution may be replaced by an asymptotic approximation. It's not surprising that much of the literature on distribution-free tests is devoted to an analysis of the permutation distributions of ranked data.

The cost of using ranks is a loss of power, that is, a diminished probability of detecting a real difference between the distributions under test. But it is not a great loss. To achieve the same power as the permutation or parametric t-test with very large samples, the Mann–Whitney test—a two-sample comparison that uses ranks in place of the original observations, requires only 3% or 4% more observations. Cheap, if the units are widgets; expensive, if the units are patients or rare Rhesus monkeys.

9.3.3. Scores

If we are testing against normal alternatives, we can improve on the power of the Mann–Whitney test by using normal scores in place of ranks.

In the general case, we replace the rank of the ith observation, r_i, say, by the expected value of the r_ith largest value in a sample of n values drawn from the distribution F, $F^{-1}[r_i/(n + 1)]$, where F is our best guess of how the observations are really distributed; (see also David [X: 1970], p. 65).

A good guess will produce an optimal test, and, sometimes, even a "bad" guess can be close to optimum. For example, Chernoff and Savage [X: 1958] show that the normal-scores test, in which ϕ is the Gaussian distribution, has a minimum asymptotic efficiency of 1 relative to the usual t-test regardlesss of the true underlying distribution.

Bell and Doksum [1965] provide detailed comparisons of the rank and normal scores tests in a variety of settings. In Bell and Doksum [1967] they provide conditions under which the normal-scores test is minimax.

Hajek and Sidak [1967] show that, in general, optimal scores for tests of location are based on the scores

$$a(j) = -\frac{f'(F^{-1}[u])}{f(F^{-1}[u])},$$

where $u = j/(N + 1)$, and f and F are the density and cumulative distribution functions, respectively, of the underlying distribution. For optimal rank tests of scale, the scores are

$$a(j) = 1 - \frac{F^{-1}[u]f'(F^{-1}[u])}{f(F^{-1}[u])}$$

9.3.4. Robust Transformations

A robust transformation preserves sample values at the center of a distribution while shrinking those in the tails. As one example [Maritz, 1981], consider

$$\phi(u) = u/(1 + u^2).$$

For u small, $\phi(u)$ is approximately u. For $u < 1$, $\phi(u)$ is a slowly increasing function of u. If we replace x_i by $\phi(x_i)$ in computing the mean, then large values will make virtually no contribution to the total.

As a second example [Huber, X: 1972], take

$$\phi(u) = (1 - \exp[-u])/(1 + \exp[-u]).$$

Again $\phi(u)$ is approximately u for u small, and is bounded between 0 and 1.

In a complex experimental design, the transformation may be applied to the residual rather than the original observation. For example, to test whether $Y = bX$, one would apply ϕ to $y' = y - bx$, rather than to y.

If you are uncertain which transformation to use, you can reduce the effect of extreme values in some cases simply by switching to a statistic based on the absolute differences $|x_i - y_i|$ in place of the squared differences $(x_i - y_i)^2$. The final choice should be dictated by your loss function (see Section 10.4).

If extreme values are unlikely, as is the case with normal alternatives, then a robust transformation will have little or no effect on the power of a test. See Maritz [1981] and Lambert [1985] for further discussion.

9.3.5. Censoring

Lambert [1985] offers a two-sample test that is both robust and powerful. First, we order the data, so that

$$X_{(1)} < \cdots < X_{(n)} \quad \text{and} \quad Y_{(1)} < \cdots < Y_{(m)}$$

To test against the alternative that the Y's are larger on the average than the X's, we replace each X_i and Y_j that is less than $k_1 = X_{(n\beta_1)}$ by k_1 and each X_i and Y_j that is greater than $k_2 = Y_{(n\beta_2)}$ by k_2, and then carry out the usual permutation test based on the sum of the observations in the first sample. Note that the censoring values are determined by the data itself. Unfortunately, there can be more than one "right" choice for β_1 and β_2, and the computations are far from straightforward. One possible compromise is to let $k_1 = X_{(2)}$ and $k_2 = Y_{(m-1)}$ for samples of fifteen or less.

9.3.6. Discarding

The most extreme method of dealing with outliers is to discard them. Although Welch and Guiterrez [1988] obtain narrower confidence intervals in matched-pairs designs through the use of permutation applied to trimmed means, there are two objections to this method. First, the resultant test is unlikely to be exact (Theorem 3.3, [Romano, 1990]). Second, discarding data reduces the power of the test. In Good [1991], I improve on the power of the Welch-Guiterrez test by treating the outliers as if they were censored. My approach is described in more detail in the next section.

9.4. Censored Data

We may not be able to make all our measurements with the same precision.

In a radioimmune assay, for example, the typical concentration curve has a sigmoidal shape with flat regions at the two extremes. In the lower, flat region of the curve, estimation is difficult, if not impossible. While binding values elsewhere may be determined to one part in a billion, in this region they merely are recorded as "below minimum."

Here is a second example: In many clinical studies, it is neither possible nor desirable to follow all patients to the end of their lifespans. Limiting the duration of the study cuts the costs of observation and puts promising new materials and processes into immediate service. But while some lifespans will be known with precision, others can be noted only as "exceeded treatment period."

In each of these examples some of the data has been censored.

9.4.1. GAMP Tests

When observations are censored, the most powerful test typically depends on the alternative, so that it is not possibie to obtain a uniformly most powerful test.

Recently [Good, 1989, 1991, 1992], I found that by establishing a region of indifference, it may be possible to obtain a permutation test that is close to the most powerful test, "almost most powerful," regardless of the underlying parameter values.

Suppose we wish to perform a test of a hypothesis F against a series of alternatives $F_1, F_2, \ldots$. To obtain a test that is globally almost most powerful (GAMP), we proceed in three stages:

First, we use the likelihood ratio to obtain a locally most powerful unbiased α-level test of the hypothesis F against the alternative F_1. We repeat this procedure for each alternative F_i to obtain a family of rejection regions $\{R_i\}$.

Next, we form two regions: (i) A rejection region $R \subseteq \bigcap_i R_i$ that contains only events common to all the rejection regions of the preceding family; and (ii) an acceptance region A that contains only events common to all the acceptance regions.

Last, we construct a permutation test whose p-value is determined by assigning each rearrangement of the data to one of three regions: rejection (R), acceptance (A), or indifference (I). While we cannot determine the p-value of their new test exactly, we can bound it:

$$\Pr\{R|X\} \le p \le 1 - \Pr\{A|X\}.$$

In Good [1992], I showed that GAMP's exist when the joint loglikelihood of the observations takes the particularly simple form $S_U * f(\theta) + N_C * g(\theta)$ where S_U and N_C are the sum of the uncensored observations and the number of censored observations in the treatment sample, respectively, and f and g are monotone functions of θ. Examples include normally distributed, exponentially distributed, and gamma distributed random variables subject to type I censoring.

A permutation (or rerandomization) approach is utilized.

There are two distinct cases, which I term left- and right-censoring respectively, though the actual directions—left or right—will depend upon the alternative. To fix ideas. suppose we have samples from two populations and are testing a null hypothesis $H: F_2 = F_1$, against stochastically larger alternatives, $K: F_2(x) = F_1(x - \delta)$. With left-censoring, we can assign x a precise value only if $x \ge c$; for example, radioimmune assay involves left-censoring. With right-censoring, we can assign x a precise value only if $x \le c$; for example, reliability studies usually involve right-censoring.

To eliminate any dependence on the zero point of the underlying scale, we transform the data before we derive the permutation distribution; from each of the orginal observations we subtract $\overline{X}_U$ the mean of the uncensored observations in the sample taken from G; $X'_{ij} = X_{ij} - \overline{X}_U$, for $i = 1, 2, j = 1, \ldots, n_i$; and $S'_{U_0} = 0$ and the transformed observations are censored at $c' = c - \overline{X}_U$. Next, we compute S_{U_0} and N_{C_0} for the original treatment sample; and permute repeatedly, computing S_U and N_C for each permuted sample.

With left-censoring, we assign a permutation to the rejection region R if $S_U \ge S_{U_0}$ and $N_C \ge N_{C_0}$. We assign it to the acceptance region A if $S_U < S_{U_0}$ and $N_C \le N_{C_0}$. We assign it to the indifference region otherwise.

With right-censoring, we impute the value c to the censored observations. Let $k = N_C - N_{C_0}$. We assign a permutation to the rejection region R if $S_U + kc \ge S_{U_0}$. We assign it to the acceptance region A if $S_U + kc < S_{U_0}$. We assign it to the indifference region otherwise.

The indifference region is small enough in most instances to permit effective decision making [Good, 1989]. As the sample size increases, the GAMP test converges in probability to a UMP unbiased test [Good, 1992]. In the rare case where the result does lie in the indifference region, I recommend taking additional observations.

The application of permutation methods to censored data was first suggested by Kalbfleisch and Prentice [1980], who sampled from the permutation distribution of censored data to obtain estimates in a process akin to bootstrapping.

For a survey of other permutation tests that have been applied to sensored data, see Schemper [1984]. Conditional rank tests for randomly censored survival data are described by Andersen et al. [1982] and Janssen [1991].

9.5. Censored Matched Pairs

As we showed in Chapter 3.6, the sensitivity of an experiment can be increased through the use of matched pairs. But it may happen that an exact observation can not be made for one or more subjects, the only available information being that the required measurement is greater or less than some known value. Often this censoring process is accidental, but in many toxicology studies and reliability trials, it is a matter of deliberate design: the experimenter trades the cost of enrolling a larger number of subjects at the onset of the experiment for a shortened study period.

Suppose $z = y - x$ is the difference between the (transformed) observations on the two members of a pair, and that observations are not recorded if they exceed C on the (transformed) scale. As noted by Sampford and Taylor [X: 1959], any pair provides information on the distribution of z in one of the following four forms:

(i) both y and x are observed, so that z is determined exactly;
(ii) x is observed, but we only know that y exceeds C; that is $z > C - x$, so we say z is upper censored;
(iii) y is observed, but we only know that x exceeds C; that is $z < y - C$, so we say z is lower censored;
(v) both x and y exceed C, so that no information is available on z for this pair; the sample size is effectively reduced.

While cases (ii) and (iii) provide less information than case (i), they are not uninformative, and a variety of hypothesis testing methods have been proposed for capitalizing on the information they provide. Recently [Good, 1991], I developed an "almost" most powerful distribution-free method based strictly on the data at hand. To see how this method is applied, assume that the first observation in each pair has the distribution F and the second has the distribution G. The hypothesis, unless stated to the contrary, is that $F \geq G$. The alternative is that $F < G$.

9.5.1. GAMP Test

The GAMP test for matched pairs represents a simple extension of the GAMP test for two independent samples derived in Good [1989, 1992]. Record U, the number of upper censored pairs in the original sample, and Z, the sum of the uncensored z's in the original sample. Randomize the observations, permuting the treatment labels within each pair, and let U' and Z' be the corresponding statistics for the permuted sample.

If $U' \geq U$ and $Z' \geq Z$, then assign the permuted sample to the rejection region R.

If $U' \leq U$ and $Z' < Z$, then assign the permuted sample to the acceptance region A.

Otherwise, assign the permuted sample to a region of indifference.

Repeat the randomization process for all possible permutations (or for a suitably large number N of randomly selected permutations) and let f_R, f_A, and f_I be the frequency with which permutations are assigned to the rejection, acceptance, and indifference regions, respectively.

This method of construction ensures that the acceptance region A of the GAMP test is contained in the acceptance regions of each of the most powerful α-level permutation tests of a simple hypothesis $G = F = F^*$ against the simple alternative $G^* = G > F = F^*$. Similarly, the rejection region R of the GAMP test is contained in the rejection regions of each of the most powerful α-level permutation tests.

$f_R \leq p \leq N - f_A$, where p is the significance level of any member of the family of most powerful permutation tests of a simple hypothesis against a simple alternative. Thus, a test of the composite hypothesis $F \leq G$ against the composite alternative $F > G$ based on the bounds defined by A and R is globally almost most powerful, or GAMP.

In practice, an investigator using a GAMP will elect one of three courses of action: 1) accept the null hypothesis, noting the bounds on the p level; 2) reject the hypothesis in favor of a stochastically larger alternative: or, 3) in order that p might be known with greater certainty, elect to take additional observations. If you require exact significance levels to make power comparisons with other tests, you must randomize on the indifference region as follows:

If f_R is greater than the desired α-level, accept the null hypothesis. If $N - f_A$ is less, reject. If neither condition holds, choose a random number $Z = U(0, 1)$ and reject the hypothesis if $Z \leq (N\alpha - f_R)/(N - f_R - f_A)$, accepting it otherwise.

9.5.2. Ranks

When data is heavily censored, you can improve on this method by replacing the original observations with ranks. Two approaches suggest themselves: In the first, which I term "post-ranking," compute the differences, z, for each pair, then rank these differences in absolute value, dividing the highest ranks among the censored observations. Denote by Z the sum of the ranks which correspond to those pairs in which y is known to be larger than x. As in the GAMP test, now randomize the observations, permuting the treatment labels within each pair, and denote by Z' the new rank sum. Assign this randomization to R, I, or A according to whether $Z' >$, $=$, or $<$ than Z. As with the GAMP test, reject H in favor of K if only a small proportion of rerandomizations are assigned to R; randomize on the indifference region I to obtain a test at a specific significance level p.

Post-ranking has the drawback that if, say, 2 is the censoring point, the difference "censored $- 1.99$" is automatically assigned a higher rank than the difference "$1.99 - 0$." To avoid this difficulty, in a second approach, which I term preranking, first rank the individual observations, again dividing the highest ranks among the censored observations. Next, compute the differences of the ranks within each pair, and, as a third and final step, rank the absolute values of the differences. The drawbacks of this second, preranked approach are computational: you must rank the data twice and you must correct for ties during the second ranking.

When the underlying distribution is normal and censoring is heavy, the preranked permutation test provides the greatest sensitivity [Good, 1991].

When the underlying distribution is normal and censoring is light, or when the underlying distribution is exponential, the GAMP test is preferable.

The strength of the GAMP lies in its use of exact values rather than ranks —thus its effectiveness with heavy-tailed distributions, like the exponential, which have many extreme values. The GAMP is also the most readily computed. Its weakness lies in its dependence on a region of indifference whose. size varies from sample to sample.

How long does it take to perform a randomization test? Using the computational shortcuts described in Section 11.3, a comparison of 15 matched pairs with complete enumeration of all rerandomizations takes twelve seconds on an 80386-based microcomputer without a floating-point coprocessor.

9.5.3. One-Sample: Bootstrap Estimates

If you are willing to assume the underlying distribution(s) are symmetric, then these methods for paired comparisons may also be applied to hypotheses based on a single sample. If censoring is one-sided, we are forced to censor on the opposite side in order to obtain an exact test. If you are unwilling to assume symmetry, and/or to throw away data through censoring, have 15 or more observations (30 would be better) and are willing to assume that all observations are drawn from the same distribution, then you may apply Efron's [X: 1981] bootstrap method of extending the Kaplan–Meir estimates.

9.6. Adaptive Tests

In an adaptive test [Hogg and Lenth, X: 1984], we compute several different test statistics, but make use only of the one we estimate to be the most powerful. For example, we could compute both a t-test and a robust test based on an M-estimate and, after the fact, use the one which seems best suited to the data. With some adaptive methods, the frequency of Type I error may increase as a result of this selection procedure. But with Donegani's method [1991] applied to two permutation tests, we can obtain a single test that is both exact and equal in power asymptotically to the most powerful of the two tests.

Let T_1, and T_2 be the two tests and let c_1, and c_2, the "criteria", be two positive real functions defined on the vector of observations X such that if $c_1(X) < c_2(X)$, then T_1 is preferable to T_2. Suppose that large values of either test statistic indicate a departure from the null hypothesis. Proceed in four steps as follows:

1. Evaluate $c_1(X), c_2(X)$ and let 'opt' refer to the index of the criterion having the smaller value.
2. Partition the set, P, of all possible rearrangements of the data into two sets

$$P_1 = \{\pi: c_1(\pi X) < c_2(\pi X)\}$$
$$P_2 = \{\pi: c_1(\pi X) > c_2(\pi X)\}$$

3. Let H_{opt} be the randomization distribution obtained by evaluating the optimal test statistic T_{opt} on each element of the set that contains the original rearrangement.

4. Reject the null hypothesis at the level α if T_{opt} exceeds the 100-αth percentile of H_{opt}. In other words, if $c_1(x) < c_2(X)$ restrict attention to those rearrangements that are in P_1.

Let N_i denote the number of rearrangements in P_i. Let C_i denote the choice of the statistic T_i. Then

$$P\{R|H\} = P\{R|H, C_1\}P\{C_1|H\} + P\{R|H, C_2\}P\{C_2|H\}$$
$$= \alpha(N_1/(N_1 + N_2)) + \alpha(N_2/(N_1 + N_2))$$
$$= \alpha.$$

Donegani [1991] shows that this adaptive procedure is asymptotically optimal and, in the case of matched pairs, that it is optimal with as few as nine pairs of observations.

9.7. Questions

1. Prove that ranking the data will eliminate any distortions brought about by a nonlinear measuring device. That is, prove that the ranks of the observations are

invariant under any continuous, strictly increasing transformation. (We take advantage of this result in a multivariate analysis in which we use ranks to bring several disparate variables together on a single common scale; see Section 5.2.)

2. Show that an exact one-sample permutation test for singly-censored data can exist only if you deliberately censor the data from the other side.

3. Let $x_1, \ldots, x_n$ be a sample from the exponential distribution with density $\frac{1}{b} e^{-x/b}$, $b > 0$. If you have a scintillation counter at hand, you can generate just such a sample by recording the time elapsed between counts. Alternately, you may stand on a street corner or at night club entrance and record the number of seconds before the next redhead or the next BMW goes by. If you have access to a computer, use its random number generator and take the logarithms of the random numbers you generate. Guesstimate the mean waiting time, b, before you start. Test your guesstimate (see Section 3.1) using a) the original observations, b) ranks, c) normal scores, and d) the data remaining after you've thrown out all observations that are three times the guesstimated value. Compare your results with the different statistical procedures for samples of size 5, 6, and 7.

CHAPTER 10

Which Statistic? Solving the Insolvable

10.1. The Permutation Distribution

Many common statistical problems defy conventional parametric analysis simply because of the distributions of the resultant test statistics are not well-tabulated. Or, worse, we settle for a less-than-optimal statistic simply because a table for the less-than-optimal statistic is readily available—the chi-square statistic (Section 6.3.1) and its misapplication to sparse contingency tables is one obvious example.

We need not settle for less than the best. Given a sufficiently powerful computer and the time needed to perform the necessary calculations, we can always obtain the permutation distribution of the statistic that best separates the hypothesis from the alternative.

The freedom of choice provided by permutation methods creates its own new set of problems. Given complete freedom in the selection of a test statistic, which statistic are we to choose?

The purpose of this chapter is two-fold: 1) to describe a number of practical applications in animal behavior, atmospheric science, education, epidemiology, molecular genetics and sociology where permutation distributions have provided new and more powerful solutions; and 2) to provide some general rules to use in the derivation of test statistics for your own demanding applications.

10.2. New Statistics

10.2.1. Nonresponders

In this section, we consider several new statistics designed specifically for use in a permutation test. An elementary example is a statistic I proposed for use when there is a response threshold, a common occurrence in pharmacological studies [Good, 1979].

We assume that $X_1, \ldots, X_n$, the controls, are independent and identically distributed with distribution F, while responders in the treatment group are independent and identically distributed as $G(x) = F(x - \delta)$. Unfortunately, not every member of the treatment group is capable of responding to the treatment; with the result that we are forced to test the hypothesis $G = F$ against contaminated alternatives of the form

$$G = pF(x - \delta) + (1 - p)F(x), \quad \text{with} \quad 0 < p \le 1 \tag{10.1}$$

The conventional statistics for the two-sample comparison—Student's t and the Wilcoxon test—are subject to a loss of power in the presence of nonresponders. This reduction in power is due to two factors: 1) a decrease in the absolute difference between the means of the two testing groups and 2) an increase in the variance of the treatment sample. This last change is the key to the selection of a new test statistic:

$$v(p) = p' \frac{nm}{(n + m)} (X. - Y.)^2 + (1 - p')S_y^2 \tag{10.2}$$

This new statistic has two components: the first is proportional to the difference $(X. - Y.)$ in the means of the two samples, the second to S_y^2, the variance of the treatment sample.

Barring the availability of an independent test for response, the p' used in equation (10.2) is at best only a guess as of the true p of equation (10.1). In Good [1979], we find that using a value of $p' = 0.67$ appears to offer relatively good protection against a broad range of values of π. Boos and Browne [1986] question whether the gain in power is really worth all the extra computation. An increase in power can mean a decrease in sample size with fewer experimental subjects placed at risk and a shortened study time with more rapid dissemination of important results. An increase in computation time puts the strain where it belongs—on the computer.

10.2.2. Animal Movement

Let $\{(w_i, x_i), i = 1, \ldots, n\}$ denote a series of paired observations on the successive positions of two organisms in space. We would like to know if the movements of the two organisms are independent or coordinated. According to Solow [1989], the ecological literature favors a test of independence based on the ratio of the actual distance travelled to the distance from the starting point:

$$R_1 = \frac{\sum \{(w_{i+1} - w_i)^2 + (x_{i+1} - x_i)^2\}}{\sum \{w_i^2 + x_i^2\}} \tag{10.3}$$

Our own intuition suggests a more powerful test of the hypothesis of independence would result from using either

$$R_2 = \frac{\sum (w_i - x_i)^2}{\sum \{w_i^2 + x_i^2\}} \tag{10.4}$$

the ratio of the successive distances of the two organisms from each other and from the starting point, or

$$R_3 = \frac{\sum (w_{i+1} - w_i)(x_{i+1} - x_i)}{\sum \{w_i^2 + x_i^2\}} \tag{10.5}$$

the traditional measure of correlation.

We also favor R_2 and R_3 on the grounds of simplicity. To compute the permutation distribution of R_1, we need to rearrange both sets of movements $\{w_i\}$ and $\{x_i\}$. To compute the permutation distribution of R_2 or R_3, we only need to rearrange one set of movements. Whatever statistic we chose, we may use its permutation distribution to obtain a test of statistical significance.

10.2.3. The Building Blocks of Life

In a fascinating state-of-the-art biological application, DNA sequencing, Karlin et al. [1983] use permutation methods to assess the significance of certain repeated patterns of nucleic acids in several viruses.

DNA, the self-replicating molecule that is the basis of life on Earth, is assembled from four specific nitrogenous bases—adenine, guanine, thymine, and cytosine. The sequence in which these bases occur in the DNA molecule determines the structure of the organism. The triplet of deoxyribonucelotides guanine-adenine-cytosine leads to the production of the amino acid aspargine, for example. At issue is whether certain repeated patterns involving multiple copies of lengthy nucleotide sequences is also significant or merely the result of chance. Studying the distribution of repeated patterns that result when one randomly reassigns the labels on the nucleotides while preserving the total numbers of each label, Karlin et al. conclude that the observed patterns are statistically significant. Hasegawa, Krishino, and Yano [X: 1988] approach an analogous problem in DNA sequencing using bootstrap methods. The unraveling of the biological significance of the patterns continues to be an important research problem.

10.2.4. Model Validation

The general circulation models of the Earth's atmosphere and oceans used in weather- and current-prediction are of mind-boggling complexity, while the

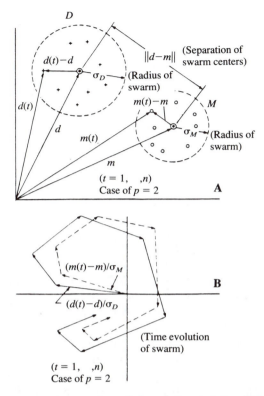

Figure 10.1. The geometric meaning of the trinity statistics SITES, SPRED and SHAPE. The statistic SITES is essentially a dimensionless measure of the separation of data swarm centroids, while SPRED is a dimensionless measure of the differences in the root-mean-square radii of the swarms. The statistic SHAPE is a combined measure of the time evolution of the data swarms (and their associated maps). Note: From "The numerical model/reality intercomposition tests using small-sample statistics," by R.W. Priesendorfer and T.P. Barnett, which appeared in *Journal of the Atmospheric Sciences*; 1983; 40: 1884–96. Reprinted with permission from the American Meteorological Society.

available data is all too finite. Priesendorfer and Barnett [1983] confront the problem of model-reality comparison studies for general circulation models head on by developing their own triple of metrics. In Figure 10.1a, and b which illustrates some of their concepts, the set D represents actual on-site data while M corresponds to a computer-generated model.

Rerandomization is accomplished in two steps. First, the data from D and M is combined into a single data set. Then, this combined set is repeatedly subdivided at random into sets of the same size as the original D and M. The resultant reference distributions for each of the three metrics are used to assess the agreement of the model with reality.

How good is the Priesendorfer-Barnett test? The answer to this question illustrates the value of the permutation approach to the scientist and engineer whose primary training is not in statistics. For the answer does not depend on the abilities of Priesendorfer and Barnett as statisticians—the calculations in their test are straightforward—but on their abilities as meteorologists and oceanographers. Their test of statistical significance will be a good one, *if* they have selected the appropriate metric and the appropriate variables.

10.2.5. Structured Exploratory Data Analysis

A further illustration of this principle is given by Karlin and Williams [1984] in their use of permutation methods in a structured exploratory data analysis (SEDA) of familial traits. A SEDA has four principal steps:

1) The data are examined for heterogeneity, discreteness, outliers, and so forth, after which they may be adjusted for covariates (as in Section 4.3) and the appropriate transform applied (as in Section 9.3).
2. A collection of summary SEDA statistics are formed from ratios of functionals.
3) The SEDA statistics are computed for the original family trait values and for reconstructed family sets formed by permuting the trait values within or across families.
4) The values of the SEDA statistics for the original data are compared with the resulting permutation distributions.

As one example of a SEDA statistic, consider the OBP, the Offspring-Between-Parent SEDA statistic:

$$\frac{\sum_{i}^{N} \sum_{j}^{K_i} |O_{ij} - (M_i + F_i)/2|}{\sum_{i}^{N} |F_i - M_i|} \tag{10.6}$$

In family $i = 1, \ldots, I$, F_i and M_i are the trait values of the father and mother (the cholesterol levels in the blood of the father and mother, for example), while O_{ij} is the trait value of the jth child, $j = 1, \ldots, K_i$.

To evaluate the permutation distribution of the OBP, we consider all permutations in which the children are kept together in their respective family units, while we either:

a) randomly assign to them a father and (separately) a mother; or
b) randomly assign to them an existing pair of spouses. The second of these methods preserves the spousal interaction. Which method we choose will depend upon the alternative(s) of interest.

It would be difficult to establish the distribution of these measures or any other SEDA statistics analytically. To obtain the permutation distribution for the OBP statistic, we merely substitute its formula (10.6) in place of the compute subroutine in our sample program (Section 4.2).

10.2.6. Comparing Multiple Methods of Assessment

We are often forced to combine several methods of assessment; one obvious example is in quality control; another is in grading students: is an "A" in statistics equivalent to an "A" in Spanish? Direct comparisons are difficult, if not impossible, when students are free to choose their own courses. Table 10.1, reproduced with permission from Manly [1988] illustrates some of the problems associated with free choice: Missing data is one obvious problem. A second, hidden problem is that there is no guarantee that a student who is good in statistics will do equally well in Spanish.

The solution to both problems is to develop some kind of aggregate measure, compute this measure separately for each course, and then check to see how the distribution of this measure is affected by random relabellings of the students.

Table 10.2, also taken from Manly, illustrates the computation of just such a measure for the course in F. (The names of the actual courses have been changed to letters to protect the identities of overly-generous and overly-stingy graders.) The students are arranged in Table 10.2 in order of increasing mean grade. Each student's mark in course F is subtracted from that student's mean grade and the differences are cumulated.

If the *marks* in the various subjects are comparable, then each random rearrangement of an individual student's marks is equally likely. For example, under the null hypothesis, student 6, who we see from Table 10.1 received marks of 75, 46, 45, and 64 in subjects A, C, E, and F might just as easily have received marks of 64, 45, 75, and 46 in those same subjects. Had this been the case, the CUMSUM score for subject F would have been 67.2 rather than 85.2. By looking at all possible arrangements of each student's marks, we obtain a permutation distribution against which the CUMSUM score for the original arrangement can be assessed.

If the original score does not represent an extreme value, we conclude that the marking for subject F is consistent with the marking for the other subjects.

If, on the other hand the original CUMSUM score does represent an extreme value, our next step is to rescale the marks for subject F, subtracting and/or dividing by a constant. We repeat the test procedure using the rescaled values. And, in a manner akin to the way in which we derive a confidence interval (see Section 3.2), we continue testing and rescaling until all the marks in all the courses have been brought into alignment. Then, we may safely combine the assessments.

Table 10.1. Examination results from seven examinations (subjects A–G) for 64 students[†]

Std	Subject							M
	A	B	C	D	E	F	G	
1	70	—	—	—	—	—	60	65.0
2	61	—	38	—	—	—	—	49.5
3	94	—	92	—	—	—	—	93.0
4	73	—	62	42	—	—	—	59.0
5	63	—	62	—	45	64	66	63.7
6	75	—	46	—	—	—	—	57.5
7	38	—	9	—	—	—	—	23.5
8	70	—	41	—	—	—	—	55.5
9	59	—	38	—	—	—	—	48.5
10	79	—	73	—	—	—	—	76.0
11	56	—	—	—	44	—	65	55.0
12	78	50	—	—	—	—	—	64.0
13	68	—	65	—	—	—	—	66.5
14	—	—	29	—	—	—	36	32.5
15	—	—	48	61	—	—	—	54.5
16	75	—	80	—	—	—	—	77.5
17	58	—	—	—	—	—	—	58.0
18	—	—	—	—	57	—	—	57.0
19	—	—	—	—	—	92	—	92.0
20	70	—	40	—	—	—	—	55.0

Std	Subject							M
	A	B	C	D	E	F	G	
33	—	—	—	—	66	51	—	58.5
34	75	—	63	67	65	—	—	67.5
35	70	—	50	—	—	—	60	60.6
36	61	59	38	—	—	—	—	53.0
37	84	—	88	—	83	42	—	78.5
38	—	—	23	28	—	—	51	32.5
39	52	—	29	—	—	—	—	40.0
40	43	—	14	—	—	—	—	28.5
41	70	—	64	—	—	—	—	67.0
42	64	—	—	—	—	—	59	61.5
43	58	—	26	—	—	—	—	42.0
44	77	—	86	—	—	—	—	81.5
45	—	—	—	—	92	—	85	88.5
46	90	—	76	—	—	—	—	83.0
47	—	—	56	43	—	—	—	49.5
48	—	—	—	—	—	—	72	72.0
49	98	94	98	94	—	—	—	96.0
50	—	85	—	95	—	—	—	90.0
51	90	—	—	—	—	—	—	90.0
52	55	—	29	—	—	—	—	42.0

Std							M
21	62	—	40	—	42	80	—	56.0
22	78	—	48	—	—	—	—	63.0
23	—	—	40	—	—	—	66	53.0
24	—	—	72	—	65	80	—	72.3
25	45	—	—	—	—	—	56	50.5
26	—	—	60	—	54	—	—	57.0
27	—	—	78	—	70	67	—	74.0
28	—	—	—	—	35	—	—	51.0
29	—	—	81	—	74	—	79	78.0
30	64	—	32	—	—	—	—	48.0
31	96	—	91	—	—	—	—	93.5
32	70	—	65	—	—	—	—	67.5

Std							M
53	65	—	39	—	—	—	—	52.0
54	60	—	—	—	—	—	—	60.0
55	—	—	52	—	58	90	—	74.0
56	90	63	84	83	—	—	—	71.0
57	91	—	92	—	—	—	—	80.3
58	90	—	41	—	—	—	—	91.0
59	64	—	1	—	—	—	—	52.5
60	20	—	26	—	—	—	—	10.5
61	45	—	79	82	—	—	—	35.5
62	91	75	56	—	—	—	—	81.8
63	60	—	—	—	—	—	—	58.0
64	—	—	—	66	—	92	—	79.0

† A dash indicates that the student concerned did not sit the examination: *Std*, student number; *M*, student mean mark.

Note: From Manly [1988]. Reprinted with permission from the Royal Statistical Society.

Table 10.2. CUSUM calculations for the subject F
marks of Table 1*

Student	F mark	Mean	Difference	CUSUM
38	42	32.5	9.5	9.5
28	67	51.0	16.0	25.5
21	80	56.0	24.0	49.5
6	64	57.5	6.5	56.0
33	51	58.5	−7.5	48.5
24	80	72.3	7.7	56.2
55	90	74.0	16.0	72.2
64	92	79.0	13.0	85.2
19	92	—	—	—

* Student 19 only took subject F. There is therefore no comparison
possible with other subjects and no contribution to the CUSUM.
Note: From "The comparison and scaling of student assessment
marks in several subjects" by B.F.J. Manly which appeared in Applied Statistics; 1988; 37: 385–95.
Note: Reprinted with permission from the Royal Statistical Society

10.3. Going Beyond

At this point, you may already be thinking about several problems of your
own for which you would like to develop an optimal test statistic. The purpose of this last section of this chapter is to provide you with the basic
principles of selection. While in Chapter 14 we consider a number of formal
derivations based on the likelihood ratio, our approach in this chapter is
more intuitive. The three essential concepts we consider are sufficiency,
invariance, and loss.

10.3.1. Sufficiency

A statistic $T(X)$ is *sufficient* for a parameter θ (or a set of parameters $\{\theta_i\}$) if
the conditional distribution of X given T is independent of θ. Once we have
calculated the value of a sufficient statistic or statistics, we may be able to
throw away the original observations, for frequently, a suffcient statistic(s)
can provide us with all the information a sample has to offer.

An example we have already encountered is that of the order statistics
$x_{(1)} \leq x_{(2)} \leq \cdots \leq x_{(n)}$. If we know these order statistics, we know as much
about the unknown distribution as we would if we had the original observa-
tions in hand.

Another commonly encountered example is that of the mean of a sample
of independent, identically Poisson-distributed random variables, a statistic
which is sufficient for the mean of the underlying Poisson distribution. Like-

wise the mean of a sample of normally-distributed random variables is sufficient for the mean of the underlying normally-distributed population. But
there is distinction: in the first example, the Poisson, the sample mean pos-
seses all the information the sample has to offer with regard to the underlying
single-parameter distribution. A normal distribution depends on two parameters, the population mean and the population variance. We need to compute
both the sample mean and the sample variance to obtain all the information
a sample from a normal distribution has to offer.

In selecting a statistic to test a hypothesis about a population parameter θ,
look first at those statistics which are sufficient for θ.

10.3.2. Invariance

If your measurements are made in feet, would you expect to reach the same
conclusions as you would if your measurements were made in inches? What
if you discover *after* you report your results that you forgot to rezero the
measurement device so that each of your readings is off by exactly 0.0123
grams. Would you still believe that your decision to accept the hypothesis is
correct? If your answers to both these questions is an unconditional "yes,"
then you are already applying the principle of invariance, implicitly if not
explicitly.

Many statistical problems involve symmetries. In the examples we've considered so far, the observations are exchangeable, so that the order in whicn
we made these observations is irrelevant. Our test statistic(s) should and
do reflect this same symmetry. The sample mean and sample variance are
good examples of statistics that are symmetric in the underlying variables.
Symmetry and invariance are related. The mathematical expression of symmetry is invariance under a suitable group of transformations. In generating
an optimal test, look for test statistics that preserve the structure and symmetry of a problem.

10.3.3. Losses

A statistical problem is defined by three elements:

1) the class $P = (P_\theta, \theta \in \Omega)$ to which the probability distribution of the observations is assumed to belong;
2) the set D of possible decisions $\{d\}$ one can make on observing $X =
   (X_1, \ldots, X_n)$,
3) the loss $L(d, \theta)$, expressed in dollars, men's lives or some other quantifiable measure, that results when we make the decision d when θ is
   true.

When you and I differ in our assessment of the loss function, we are likely to differ in our assessment of the practical significance of Type I and Type II error and, hence, in our choice of test statistic.

The loss function should be a key factor in the selection of a statistical test. Even when we don't know the exact values taken by a loss function, we have some idea about its form. In many testing situations, for example, in the analysis of variance and in some matched pair applications, the traditional test statistic (or discrepancy measure in Mehta and Patel's terminology) is a function of the square of the distance between the observed or estimated values and the hypothesis. Yet the natural measure is the distance itself. A statistical procedure that minimizes the expected value of the one may not minimize the expected value of the other [Mielke and Berry, 1982, 1983].

The principal reason for using the square of the distance is that it yields a maximum likelihood solution when the underlying distribution is normal. An assumption of normality may or may not be justified while maximum likelihood itself can only be justified on the grounds of convenience.

A second and more compelling reason for using the square of the distance in the data space would be that the loss function, a discrepancy measure in the parameter space, is also proportional to the square. But if we are uncertain about the form of the loss function, wouldn't it be more natural to utilize a test statistic that is linear in both the data and parameter spaces? A first-order statistic will be more robust than a second-order statistic in the face of questionably large deviations [Dodge, 1987].

The permutation approach frees us to choose the test statistic that is best suited to the problem at hand. If a second-order statistic is called for, we may use it, and if a first-order statistic is more appropriate, we may take advantage of it instead. Through the use of resampling methods we are free to choose the statistic best suited to the problem.

Recall from Section 4.2 that if we have more than two levels of a factor, we have a choice of at least three test statistics:

$$F2 = \sum_{j=1}^{J} \sum_{k=1}^{K} \sum_{i=1}^{I} n_{ijk}(X_{ijk\cdot} - X_{\cdot jk\cdot})^2 \qquad (10.7)$$

a second-order statistic;

$$F1 = \sum_{j=1}^{J} \sum_{k=1}^{K} \sum_{i=1}^{I} n_{ijk}|X_{ijk\cdot} - X_{\cdot jk\cdot}| \qquad (10.8)$$

a first-order statistic; and

$$R = \sum_{j=1}^{J} \sum_{k=1}^{K} \sum_{i=1}^{I} n_{ijk}f[i](X_{ijk\cdot} - X_{\cdot jk\cdot}) \qquad (10.9)$$

With the permutation approach, we are free to select the optimal statistic in accordance with both the alternatives of interest and the underlying loss function.

10.4. Likelihood Ratio

As we shall see in Chapter 14.2, the primary criteria for selecting a test statistic is the likelihood ratio. We assign to our acceptance region those values of our test statistic for which the likelihood under the hypothesis is much greater than it is under the alternative and to the rejection region those values which are much more likely under the alternative than they are under the hypothesis.

To see this intuitively, suppose the variables can take only a countable number of values, $P_i\{X = x\} = p_i(x)$ for $i = 0, 1, \dots$.

The optimal test is obtained by finding a set of values S to form the rejection region for which the significance level

$$\sum_{x \in S} p_0(x) \leq \alpha \tag{10.10}$$

and the power

$$\sum_{x \in S} p_1(x) \text{ is a maximum.} \tag{10.11}$$

Which values of x should we include in S? Clearly, we should include those values which contribute the least to the significance level while contributing the most to the power. In other words, we should include those values of x with the largest values of the likelihood ratio

$$r(x) = \frac{p_1(x)}{p_0(x)}. \tag{10.12}$$

We extend this result to continuous distribution functions in Section 14.2 with the fundamental lemma of Neyman and Pearson.

The cutoff—that is, the precise definition of "largest" values—is determined by the significance level. Using the likelihood ratio, we show in Chapter 14 that the same criteria which led to the t-statistic and the F-ratio for the parametric analysis of two and k samples, respectively, leads to the use of statistics equivalent to the t and the F-ratio for the corresponding permutation analyses. In Chapter 6.2, the likelihood ratio is used to derive Fisher's exact test and to show that it is the most powerful unbiased test we can use with a 2×2 contingency table.

10.4.1. Goodness of Fit and the Restricted Chi-Square

In the next example, that of an $r \times 1$ contingency table. we can not derive a most powerful test that will protect us against all alternatives, but we can use the likelihood ratio to derive a most powerful test against those alternatives which are of immediate interest. The approach lends itself to any set of data for which we have knowledge of an underlying model.

Suppose the hypothesis to be tested is that certain events (births, deaths, accidents) occur randomly over a given time interval. If we divide this time interval into m equal parts and p_i denotes the probability of an event in the ith subinterval, the null hypothesis becomes $H: p_i = 1/m$ for $i = 1, \ldots, m$. Our test statistic is

$$\chi^2 = mn \sum_{i=1}^{m} \left(v_i - \frac{1}{m} \right)^2,$$

where v_i is the relative frequency of occurrence in the ith interval.

0	1	2	3	$n-1$
v_0	v_1			v_{n-1}

To determine whether this test statistic is large, small, or merely average, we examine the distribution of χ^2 for all sets of frequencies $\{v_i\}$ that satisfy the two conditions

1) $v_i \geq 0$ $i = 1, \ldots, m$; and
2) $\sum v_i = 1$.

We reject the hypothesis if the fraction of tables for which $\chi^2 \leq \chi_0^2$ is less than α.

We can obtain a still more powerful test when we know more about the underlying model and, thus, are able to focus on a narrower class of alternatives.

Suppose, in contrast to the previous example, that we use the m categories to record the results of n repetitions of a series of $m - 1$ trials, that is, we let the ith category correspond to the number of repetitions which result in exactly $i - 1$ successes. If our hypothesis is that the probability of success is .5 in each individual trial, then the expected number of repetitions resulting in exactly k successes is $\pi_k[.5] = n\binom{m}{k}(.5)^m$.

If we proceed as we did in the preceding example, then our test statistic would be

$$S_1 = \chi^2 = n \sum_{k=1}^{m} \frac{(v_k - \pi_k[.5])^2}{\pi_k[.5]} \tag{10.13}$$

Such a test provides us with protection against a wide variety of alternatives. But from the description of the problem we see that we can restrict ourselves to alternatives for which

$$\pi_k[p] = n\binom{m}{k}(p)^k(1 - p)^{m-k}. \tag{10.14}$$

Fix, Hodges, and Lehmann [X: 1959] show that a more powerful test statistic against such alternatives is

$$S = S_1 - S_2,$$

where

$$S_2 = \min_{p} \sum_{i=1}^{m} \frac{(v_i - p_i[p])^2}{\pi_i[p]} \tag{10.15}$$

The parametric form of the distribution of S is difficult if not impossible to obtain analytically except for very large sample sizes; as always, the permutation distribution is readily computed.

10.4.2. Censored Data

In Section 9.5, we use the likelihood ratio to derive a globally almost powerful test for use with censored data.

Kalbfleish and Prentice [1980] also use the likelihood ratio to obtain tests for use against highly specific alternatives when the underlying distributions are censored. The calculations are complex, so these authors suggest *bootstrapping* from the permutation distribution as a computational shortcut. Their test is appropriate when the parameters of the alternative are known with some precision. Against global and unspecified alternatives, the GAMP test described in Section 9.5 is to be preferred.

10.4.3. Logistic Regression

Finally, we use the likelihood ratio to derive a procedure which is of inestimable value in the analysis of epidemiological data. One of the earliest applications of logistic regression is that of Pike, Casagrande and Smith [1975]. For each subject, we have a pair of observations, x_i the length of exposure and y_i the apparent effect, where y_i may be a vector of several variables. To eliminate extraneous variation, we divide the data into blocks based on age, duration of residence, marital status, and so forth. Each block may be further subdivided into two not necessarily equal-sized groups—cases and controls. We would like to know if the risk of exposure is the same for each group and to estimate the relative risk.

Following Breslow and Day [1980, 1987], we condition the likelihood of x given y on the set of exposures without regard to which are cases and which are controls.

$$\frac{\prod_{j=1}^{n} L(x_j|y_j = 1) \prod_{j=1}^{m} L(x_j|_j = 0)}{\sum_{\pi \in R} \prod_{j=1}^{n} L(x_{\pi(j)}|y_j = 1) \prod_{j=1}^{m} L(x_{\pi(j)}|y_j = 0)} \tag{10.16}$$

where R is the set of $\binom{n+m}{n}$ possible reassignments π of case labels to subjects and the likelihood

$$L(x|y) = \frac{pr(y|x)pr(x)}{pr(y)}$$

Assume that within a block, the observations satisfy the logistic regression model, so that

$$pr\{y|x\} = \frac{\exp[\alpha + \beta x]}{1 + \exp[\alpha + \beta x]}$$

The conditional likelihood (10.1) reduces to

$$\frac{\prod_{j=1}^{n} \exp\left[\sum_{k=0}^{1} \beta_k x_{\pi(j)k}\right]}{\sum_{\pi \in R} \prod_{j=1}^{n} \exp\left[\prod_{k=0}^{1} \beta_k x_{\pi(j)k}\right]} \tag{10.17}$$

an expression which depends only on the relative risk parameters β_0 and β_1.

10.5. Questions

1. Suppose you wish to compare two groups of observations. Would it be better to compare them using the two-sample comparison of Section 3.3 or the matched pairs technique of 3.6? Is your decision rule an "always ..." or does it depend on how the observations are dispersed and the relative importance of the co-variates used to do the matching?

2. Suppose you have discarded the n original observations in the sample, keeping only the n order statistics, when you obtain independent evidence that the data is normally distributed: can you still compute the sample mean and variance?

3. Suppose you have multiple observations on each subject, some in feet, some in inches, some in pounds. Should they all be transformed to a common unit of reference before you begin your multivariate analysis? What transformation(s) should you use?

4. What statistic(s) remain invariant under an arbitrary monotone increasing transformation of the observations? Is this result relevant to the preceding question?

5. Ninety-nine percent of all scientists ignore the loss function and make do with a predesignated significance level and a minimum power level against one or two selected alternatives. Reconsider the statistical analyses you performed recently. What was the loss function in each instance? Were the test statistics you selected appropriate for this loss function?

6. a. Can the four k-sample statistics, F1, F2, F3, and R introduced in Section 4.2.2 be made equivalent to one another if we eliminate terms that are invariant under permutations?
   b. If your answer to the previous question is "no," will there be data sets for which tests based on F1, F2, and R lead to different conclusions?

c. How would you decide which of these statistics to use?

d. Are you free to compute the permutation distributions of F1, F2, and R for a specific data set and then choose the statistic which does the best job of proving your point?

e. Suppose you were an examiner at the FDA; how would you react to a submission the authors of which had done just that?

f. If you were one of those authors, how would you justify your choice of test statistic to an examiner at the FDA?

g. Throughout this text, we have tried to justify our choice of statistic on the grounds that the resuitant test was a) unbiased, b) most powerful, c) minimized losses, or was d) invariant under transformations of location and scale. Do these criteria satisfy your own instincts? What other criteria can you suggest?

Which Test Should You Use?

In this chapter we provide you with an expert system for use in choosing an appropriate testing technique. Your expert system comes to you in two versions—a professional's handbook with detailed explanations of the choices, and a short, "quick-reference" version at the end of the chapter.

11.1. Sources of Variation

A few preliminary definitions are required. First, we distinguish a parametric from a nonparametric test:

To perform a parametric test, we must assume the observations come from a probability distribution which has a specific parametric form. For example, an observation, X, has the Poisson distribution with parameter λ if the probability that $X = k$ is $\lambda^k \exp[-\lambda]/k!$ for $k = 0, 1, 2, \ldots$. An observation, X, has the normal distribution with location parameter μ and scale parameter σ if the probability density, $h(x)$, is

$$\frac{1}{\sqrt{2\pi\sigma}} \exp\left[-\frac{(x-\mu)^2}{2\sigma^2}\right].$$

While there exist various techniques for verifying whether a set of observations does or does not have a Poisson or normal distribution, the following heuristic definitions have proved of great value in practice:

An observation has the Poisson distribution if it is the cumulative result of a large number of opportunities each of which has only a small chance of occurring. For example, if we seed a small number of cells into a petri dish that is divided into a large number of squares, the distribution of cells per square follows the Poisson.

An observation has the Gaussian, or normal, distribution if it is the sum of a large number of factors—each of which makes a very small contribution to the total. This explains why the mean of a large number, N, of observations, $X. = \sum_{j=1}^{N} X_j/N$, will be normally distributed even if the individual observations X_j come from quite different distributions.

By contrast, proportions and the ratios of variables or sums of variables seldom have a normal distribution.

In many applications in economics and pharmacology where changes are often best expressed in percentages, a variable may be the product of a large number of variables each of which makes only a near unit contribution to the total. Such a variable has the lognormal distribution and, because $\log \prod x_i = \sum \log(x_i)$, its logarithm has a normal distribution.

The normal distribution is easy to recognize. It is symmetrically distributed about the mean and falls off rapidly in the tails so there is only a small probability of observing extremely large or extremely small values.

Many other distributions one encounters in practice—chi-square, Beta, Student's t and the F-ratio are all examples—may be derived from variables which have the normal distribution. For example, if X has the normal distribution with mean 0 and variance σ^2 then $Y = (X/\sigma)^2$ has the chi-square distribution with one degree of freedom.

Gamma distributions,

$$f(x|a, b) = \frac{1}{\Gamma(a)b^a} x^{a-1} e^{-x/b}$$

come into existence in complex systems where the failure of several simple parallel components is necessary before the system fails to function.

The literature is replete with methods for determining whether observations are normally distributed. My own preference is to use a nonparametric test and, preferably, a permutation test whenever there is the slightest doubt as to the nature of the underlying distribution.

Of course, one may use a parametric test when:

1) You have a large number of observations (≥ 20) in each category; or
2) You have a very small number of observations in each category and the assumptions underlying the corresponding parametric test may be relied on.

For example, if we have only three observations with which to test the hypothesis that the mean of a symmetric distribution is zero, the sample space for the permutation test is limited to 2^3 or 8 rerandomizations. As a result, we must randomize on the boundary except for significance levels that are multiples of 1/8th. At all significance levels, a more powerful parametric test, and (if we may rely on the normality of the observations) a uniformly most powerful unbiased parametric test may be obtained directly from tables of the t-statistic.

11.2. Comparison with the Parametric Test and the Bootstrap

These caveats aside, in most practical testing situations, we would advise the reader to use a permutation test or, at least, to use the permutation distribution in place of the parametric distribution:

The permutation test is exact under relatively nonstringent conditions: in the one-sample problem, the variables must have symmetric distributions; in the two- and k-sample problem, the variables must be exchangeable among the samples.

The permutation test provides protection against deviations from parametric assumptions, yet it is usually as powerful as the corresponding unbiased parametric test even for small samples.

With two binomial or two Poisson populations, the most powerful unbiased permutation test and the most powerful parametric test coincide. With two normal populations, the most powerful unbiased permutation test and the most powerful unbiased parametric test are asymptotically equivalent.

Using the permutation test means you can choose the statistic that is best adapted to your problem and to the alternatives of interest.

Consider a permutation test before you turn to a bootstrap. The bootstrap is not exact except for quite large samples and, often, is not very powerful. But the bootstrap can sometimes be applied when the permutation test fails: one example is interaction in an unbalanced design (Section 4.4) for which neither an exact parametric test nor an exact permutation test can be formulated.

11.3. A Guide to Selection

The initial division of this guide is into three groupings: categorical data, discrete data, continuous data.

11.3.1. The Data Is in Categories

Examples include men vs. women, white vs. black vs. Hispanic vs. other; and much improved vs. improved vs. no change vs. worse vs. much worse.

Only a single factor is involved.
    You are testing the goodness of fit of a specific model. See Section 10.4.1.
Only two factors are involved. For example, sex vs. political party.
    Each factor is at exactly two levels.

There is a single table.

Use Fisher's exact test (see Section 6.2).

There are several 2 × 2 tables.

Use odds' ratio test (see Section 6.2.2).

One factor is at three or more levels.

This factor is not ordered as would be the case with a factor like race.

You want a test that provides protection against a broad variety of alternatives.

Use the permutation distribution of the chi-square statistic (section 6.3.1).

You wish to test against the alternative of a cause-effect dependence.

Use the permutation distribution of τ (Freeman and Halton, 1958; see Section 6.3.1 for other possible tests).

This factor can be ordered.

Use Pitman correlation (see Section 3.5).

Both factors are at three or more levels.

Neither factor can be ordered.

The alternative is that the first factor is caused or affected by the other.

Use the permutation distribution of Kendall's tau or Cochran's Q (see Section 6.3).

A cause and effect relationship is not suspected.

Use the permutation distribution of the chi-square statistic (see Section 6.3).

One factor can be ordered.

Assign scores to this factor based on your best understanding of its effects on the second variable.

All the odds ratios are approximately equal.

Use λ_3 or the Goodman-Kruskal test (see Section 6.4).

Some but not all of the odds ratios are close to one.

Use λ_2 or the likelihood ratio test (see Chapter 6, Section 4).

A third covariate factor is present.

Use the method of Bross [1964]. See Section 6.5.

11.3.2. The Data Is Discrete, Taking the Values from the Finite Set 0, 1, ..., n or the Infinite Set 0, 1, 2, ...

Each sample consists of a fixed number of independent identically distributed observations which can be either 0 or 1. (A set of trials each of which may result in a success or a failure is one example.)

Only one or two samples are involved.

Use the parametric test for the binomial. See for example, Lehmann, [1986] pp. 81, 154.

More than two samples, but only one factor is involved.
    Analyze as indicated above under categorical data.
More than one factor is involved.
    Transform the data to equalize the variances. For each factor combi-
    nation, take the arcsin of the square root of the proportion of observa-
    tions that take the value 1. Analyze the results as indicated below
    under continuous data.
Each sample consists of a set of independent identically distributed Pois-
son observations.
    Only one or two samples are involved.
        Use the parametric test for the Poisson. In the two-sample case, note
        that the UMPU test uses the binomial distribution. See for example,
        Lehmann [1986, pp. 81, 152].
    More than two samples are involved.
        Transform the data to equalize the variances by taking the square
        root of each observation. Analyze as indicated below under continu-
        ous data.
Each sample consists of a set of exchangeable observations whose distribution is unknown.
    There is a single sample.
        The data may be assumed to come from a symmetric distribution.
            Use the permutation test for a location parameter that is described
            in Chapter 3.1.
        The data may not be assumed to come from a symmetric distribution.
            Use the bootstrap described in Section 3.4. If you have only a few
            subjects, consider using a multivariate approach (see Chapter 5).
    There is more than one sample.
        Use one of the permutation tests designed for data with continuous
        distributions that is described in Chapters 3 and 4. Treat tied obser-
        vations as separate distinct observations when you form rearrange-
        ments. Be cautious in interpreting a negative finding; the significance
        level may be too large simply because the test statistic can take on too
        few distinct values.

11.3.3. The Data Is Continuous

How precise do our measurements have to be so that we may categorize
them as "continuous" rather than discrete? Should they be accurate to two
decimal places as in 1.02? or four as in 1.0203? To apply statistical procedures
for continuous variables, the observations need only be precise enough that
there are no or only a very few ties.

If you recognize that the data has the normal distribution,
    a parametric test like Student's t or the F-ratio may be applicable. But

you can protect yourself against deviations from normality by making use of a permutation test based on the t statistic or the F.

You have only a single sample.

You want to test that the location parameter has a specific value.

And you feel safe in assuming that the underlying distribution is symmetric about the location parameter.

Use the procedure described in Section 3.1.

If the distribution is not symmetric,

but has a known parametric form

apply the corresponding parametric test;

and does not have a known parametric form,

consider applying an initial transformation that will symmetrize the data. For example, take the logarithm of data that undergoes percentage changes. Be warned that such a transformation affects the form of the loss function.

and/or bootstrap (see Section 3.4).

You want to test that the scale parameter has a specific value.

First, divide each observation by the hypothesized value of the scale parameter. Then, apply one of the procedures noted above for testing a location parameter.

You have two samples.

You want to test whether the scale parameters of the two populations are equal.

You know the means/medians of the two populations or you know that they are equal.

Use the permutation-distribution of the F-ratio based on the sample variances (see Section 3.3.2).

You have no information about the means/medians of the two populations.

The sample sizes are equal.

Use the pivot-permutation test (Section 3.4).

Sample sizes are not equal.

Use the bootstrap (Section 3.4).

You want to test whether the location parameters of the two populations are equal.

If changes are proportional rather than additive, consider working with the logarithms of the observations.

If the data is censored or you suspect outliers, see Chapter 9.

Each sample consists of measures taken on different subjects.

Use the two-sample comparison described in Section 3.3.

Two observations were made on each subject; these observations are to be compared.

Use the matched-pair comparison described in Chapter 3, Sections 1 and 6.

You have more than two samples
  If changes are proportional rather than additive, consider working with
  the logarithms of the observations.
  If the data is censored or you suspect outliers, see Chapter 9.
  A single factor distinguishes the various samples.
    You can't take advantage of other factors to block the samples.
      The factor levels are not ordered.
        Use the permutation distribution of an F-ratio (see Section 3.5).
      The factor levels are ordered.
        Use Pitman's correlation (Section 3.5.2).
    You can take advantage of other factors to block the samples.
      Rerandomize on a block-by-block basis, then apply one of the tech-
      niques described in Sections 3.6 and 3.7.
  Multiple factors are involved.
    One of the factors consists of repeated measurements made over time.
      Treat the repeated measurements as components of a single multi-
      variate vector. See Section 5.5.
    All observations are exchangeable.
      The experimental design is balanced.
        All the factors are under your control.
          Use one of the permutation techniques described in Section 4.2.
        Not all the factors are under your control.
          First, correct for the functional relation-ship among factors or
          use restricted randomization as described in Section 4.3, then,
          use one of the permutation techniques described in Section 4.2.
      The experimental design is not balanced.
        Some factors will be confounded. A book on experimental de-
        sign such as that of Kempthorne [1952], can help you determine
        which factors. Consider the bootstrap (see Section 4.4.2).

11.4. Quick Key

Categorical Data

Single factor, $r = 1$
  Goodness of fit, 10.4.1.
Two factors, $r = 2$
  $c = 2$
    single table
      use Fisher's exact test, 6.2
    several 2×2 tables
      use Zelen's exact test, 6.2.2

$c > 2$.
    not ordered
        use C^2 or τ, 6.3
    ordered
        use Pitman correlation, 3.5.
Two factors, $r > 2, c > 2$
    not ordered
        use $\tau, Q \Rightarrow 6.2, 6.3$
    ordered
        use λ_2 or λ_3, 6.4
    with covariate
        use Bross method, 6.5.

Discrete Data

Binomial Data
    one factor, one or two samples
        see Lehmann [1986, pp. 81, 154]
        one factor, more than two samples
            see categorical data
    more than one factor
        see continuous data.
Poisson data
    one or two samples.
        see Lehmann [1986, pp. 81, 152]
    more than two samples
        see under continuous data.
Other exchangeable observations
    one sample.
        symmetric distribution
        See 3.1
        not symmetric
        use bootstrap
    more than one sample
    transform data; see under continuous data.

Continuous Data

One sample
    test of location parameter
        symmetric distribution
        See 3.1

    not symmetric
        attempt to transform to some known parametric or symmetric
        form
    test of scale parameter
    rescale and test as for location parameter.
Two samples
    test equality of scale parameters
        means/medians of the two populations are known or
        are known to be equal
            F-ratio of the sample variances, 3.3.2
        otherwise
            permute or bootstrap, 3.4
    test equality of location parameters
        samples not matched
            two-sample comparison, 3.3
        samples are matched
            matched-pair comparison, 3.7, 3.1.
More than two samples
    single factor
        no blocking
            levels not ordered
                F-ratio, 3.5
            levels ordered
                Pitman correlation, 3.5.2
        blocks
            resample block by block, 3.6, 3.7
    multiple factors
        repeated measures
            muitivariate analysis, 5.5
        independent observations
            balanced design
                all factors under your control, 4.2
                otherwise, correct as in 4.3,
                then apply 4.2
            unbalanced design
                consult text on experimental design; consider bootstrap 4.4.2.

CHAPTER 12

Publishing Your Results

McKinney et al. [1989] report that more than half the published articles that apply Fisher's exact test do so improperly. Our own survey of some fifty biological and medical journals supports their findings. This chapter provides you with a positive prescription for the successful application and publication of the results of resampling procedures. First, we consider the rules you must follow to ensure that your data can be analyzed by statistical and permutation methods. Then, we describe two commercially-available computer programs that can perform a wide variety of permutation analyses. Finally, we provide you with five simple rules to prepare your report for publication.

12.1. Design Methodology

It's never too late to recheck your design methodology. Recheck it now in the privacy of your office rather than before a large and critical audience. All hypothesis-testing methods rely on the independence and/or the exchangeability of the observations. Were your observations independent of one another? What was the experimental unit? Were your subjects/plots assigned at random to treatment? If not, how was randomization restricted? With complex multifactor experiments, you need to list the blocking variables and describe your randomization scheme.

12.1.1. Randomization in Assignment

Are we ever really justified in exchanging labels among observations? Consider an experiment in which we give six different animals exactly the same treatment. Because of inherent differences among the animals, we end up with six different measurements, some large, some small, some in between. Suppose we arbitrarily label the first three measurements as "controls" and the last three as "treatment." These arbitrary labels are exchangeable and thus the probability is one in 20 that the three "control" observations will all be smaller than the three "treatment." Now suppose we repeat the experiment, only this time we give three of the animals an experimental drug and three a saline solution. To be sure of getting a positive result, we give the experimental drug to those animals who got the three highest scores in the first experiment. Not fair, you say. Illegal! Illegitimate! No one would ever do this in practice.

In the very first set of clinical data that was brought to me for statistical analysis, a young surgeon described the problems he was having with his chief of surgery. "I've developed a new method for giving arteriograms which I feel can cut down on the necessity for repeated amputations. But my chief will only let me try out the technique on patients that he feels are hopeless. Will this affect my results?" It would and it did. Patients examined by the new method had a very poor recovery rate. But, of course, the only patients who'd been examined by the new method were those with a poor prognosis. The young surgeon realized that he would not be able to test his theory until he was able to assign patients to treatment at random.

Not incidentally, it took us three more tries until we got this particular experiment right. In our next attempt, the chief of surgery—Mark Craig of St Eligius in Boston—announced that he would do the "random" assignments. He finally was persuaded to let me make the assignment using a table of random numbers. But then he announced that he, and not the younger surgeon, would perform the operations on the patients examined by the traditional method to make sure "they were done right." Of course, this turned a comparison of methods into a comparison of surgeons and intent.

In the end, we were able to create the ideal "double blind" study: the young surgeon performed all the operations, but the incision points were determined by his chief after examining one or the other of the two types of arteriogram.

12.1.2. Choosing the Experimental Unit

The exchangeability of the observations is a sufficient condition for a permutation test to be exact. It is also a necessary condition for the application of any statistical test.

Suppose you were to study several pregnant animals that had been inadvertently exposed to radiation (or acid rain or some other undesirable pollutant) and examine their offspring for birth defects. Let X_{ij} $i = 1, \ldots, l; j = 1, \ldots, n_i$ denote the number of defects in the jth offspring of the ith parent; let $Y_i = \sum_{j=1}^{n_i} X_{ij}$ $i = 1, \ldots, l$ denote the number of defects in the ith litter. The $\{Y_i\}$

may be exchangeable; (we would have to know more about how the data were collected). The $\{X_{ij}\}$ are not; the observations within a litter are interdependent; what affects a parent affects all her offspring. In this experiment, the litter is the correct experimental unit.

In a typical toxicology study, a pathologist may have to examine three to five slides at each of fifteen to twenty sites in each of three to five animals just to get a sample size of *one*.

12.2. Statistical Software for Exact Distribution-Free Inference

StatXact® uses the algorithms developed by Mehta and Patel to help perform a wide variety of permutation tests for one and two samples, $R \times C$ contingency tables, and stratified 2×2 and $2 \times C$ contingency tables. The two-sample procedures include stratified linear rank tests, Wilcoxon-Mann-Whitney test, logrank and Wilcoxon-Gehan tests for censored survival data, normal scores test, and trend test with equally spaced scores. The manual incorporates many excellent examples from the literature.

LogXact® performs exact logistic regressions as described in Cox [1970]. (*StatXact* and *LogXact* are available for IBM-PC compatible microcomputers from Cytel Software, 137 Erie St, Cambridge MA 02139. 617/661–2011.)

Most commercially available statistical packages have some provision for running Fisher's exact test in the analysis of a 2×2 contingency table. "Proc Freq" in *SAS*® uses the Mehta-Patel network algorithm to obtain exact rejection levels for $R \times C$ contingency tables.

RT® performs permutation tests on one- and two-samples (though fewer than can be done in *StatXact*), plus analysis of variance, regression analysis, matrix randomization tests, tests on spatial data, time series analysis, and multivariate analysis using Wilk's lambda statistic and Romesburg's sum of squares statistic E. Applications are drawn from Manly [1991]. (*RT* is available for IBM-PC compatible microcomputers from West, 1406 South Greeley Highway, Cheyenne WY 82007. 307/634-1756.)

12.3. Preparing Manuscripts for Publication

You've laid the groundwork. You've done the experiment. You've completed the analysis. Five simple rules can help you prepare your article for publication:

1. State the test statistic explicitly. Reproduce the formulae. If you cite a text, for example, [Good, 1994], include the page number(s) on which the statistic you are using is defined.

2. State your assumptions. Are your observations independent? Exchange-able? Is the underlying distribution symmetric? Permutation tests can not be employed without one or all of these essential assumptions.

3. State which labels you are rearranging. Provide enough detail that any interested reader can readily reproduce your results. In other words, re-port your statistical procedures in the same detail you report your other experimental and survey methodologies.

4. State whether you are using a one-tailed or a two tailed-test. See Chapter 6, Section 2 for help in making a decision.

5. a) If you detect a statistically significant effect, then provide a confidence interval (see Section 3.2). Remember: an effect can be statistically signi-ficant without being of practical or scientific significance.

   b) If you do not detect a statistically significant effect, could a larger sample or a more sensitive experiment have detected one? Consider reporting the power of your test. (See Section 13.7.)

CHAPTER 13

Increasing Computational Efficiency

13.1. Five Techniques

With today's high-speed computers, drawing large numbers of subsamples with replacement (the bootstrap) or without (the permutation test) is no longer a problem; unless and until the entire world begins computing resampling tests. To prepare for this eventuality, and because computational efficiency is essential in the search for more powerful tests, a secondary focus of research in resampling today is the development of algorithms for rapid computation.

There are five main computational approaches, several of which may be and usually are employed in tandem:

1. The *Monte Carlo*, in which a sample of the possible rearrangements is drawn at random and these samples are used in place of the complete permutation distribution.
2. *Rapid enumeration and selection algorithms*, whose object is to provide a rapid transition from one rearrangement to the next.
3. *Branch and bound algorithms* that eliminate the need to evaluate each individual rearrangement.
4. Solutions through *characteristic functions* and *fast Fourier transforms*.
5. *Asymptotic approximations*, for use with sufficiently large samples.

In the following sections, we consider each of these approaches in turn.

13.2. Monte Carlo

Instead of examining all possible rearrangements, we can substantially reduce the computations required by examining only a small but representative random sample [Dwass, 1957; Barnard, 1963]. In this process, termed a "Monte Carlo," we proceed in stages:

1) We rearrange the data at random.
2) We compute the test statistic for the rearranged data and compare its value with that of the statistic for the original sample.
3) We apply a stopping rule to determine whether we should continue sampling, or whether we are already in a position to accept or reject.

The program fragments reproduced in Chapters 3–5 of this text use the Monte Carlo approach. In the not necessarily optimal computer algorithm introduced in those chapters, all the observations in all the subsamples are loaded into a single linear vector, $X = \{X[0], X[1], \ldots, X[N-1]\}$. Then, a random number is chosen from the set of integers $0, 1, \ldots, l$ with $l = N - 1$ initially. If the number we choose is i, $X[i]$ is swapped with $X[l]$ in a three-step process:

$$\text{temp} := X[i];$$

$$X[i] := X[l-1];$$

$$X[l-1] := \text{temp};$$

and l is decremented. This process is repeated until we have rearranged the desired number of observations and are ready to compute the test statistic for the new rearrangement.

We don't always need to reselect all N observations. For example, in a two-sample comparison of means, with $N = n + m$, our test statistic only makes use of the last m observations. Consequently, we only need to choose m random numbers each time.

After we obtain the new value of the test statistic we compare it with the value obtained for the original data. We continue until we have examined N random rearrangements and N values of the test statistic. Typically, N is assigned a value between 100 and 1600 depending on the precision that is desired (see Section 13.2.2 and Marriott [1979]). Through the use of a Monte Carlo, even the most complicated multivariate experimental design can be analyzed in less than a minute on a desktop computer.

13.2.1. Stopping Rules

If a simple accept/reject decision is required, we needn't perform all N calculations, but can stop as soon as it is obvious that we must accept or reject the hypothesis at a specific level. In practice, I use a one-sided stopping rule based on the 10% level. Suppose in the first n rearrangements, we observe a fraction $H(n)$ with a value of the test statistic that is as or more extreme than the value for the original observations. If $H(n) > 0.1N$, then we accept the hypothesis at the 10% level. Otherwise, we continue until $n = N$ and report the exact percentage of rejections. Besag and Clifford [1991] and Lock [1991] describe two-sided sequential procedures in which the decision to accept, reject, or continue is made after each rearrangement is examined.

13.2.2. Variance of the Result

The resultant estimated significance level $\hat{p}$ is actually a binomial random variable $B(N, p)$, where N is the number of random rearrangements and p is the true but still unknown value of the significance level. The variance of $\hat{p}$ is $p(1 - p)/N$. If p is 10%, then using a sample of 81 randomly selected rearrangements provides a standard deviation for $\hat{p}$ is of 1%. A sample of 364 reduces the standard deviation to 0.25%.

The use of a variable in place of a fixed significance level results in a minor reduction in the power of the test particularly with near alternatives [Dwass, 1957]. In most cases, this reduction does not appear to be of any practical significance; see Vadiveloo [1983]; Jockel [1986]; Bailer [1989]; Edgington [1987]; and Noreen [1989].

13.2.3. Cutting the Computation Time

The generation of random rearrangements creates its own set of computational problems.

Each time a data element is selected for use in the test statistic, two computations are required: 1) a random number is selected; and 2) two elements in the combined sample are swapped.

The ideal futuristic computer will have a built-in random number generator—for example, it might contain a small quantity of a radioactive isotope, with the random intervals between decays producing a steady stream of random numbers. This futuristic computer might also have a butterfly network that would randomly swap ten or one hundred elements of an array in a single pass.

Today, in the absence of such technology, any improvements in computation speed must be brought about through software. Little direct research has been done in the area, although recently Baglivo et al. [1992] reported on techniques for doing many of the repetitive computations in parallel. I did some preliminary work in which I considered a sort of drunkard's walk through the set of rearrangements: the first rearrangement was chosen at random; thereafter the program stumbled from rearrangement to rearrangement swapping exactly two data elements at random each time. The results were disappointing. Any savings in computation time per rearrangement were more than offset by the need to sample four or five times as many rearrangements to achieve the same precision in the result.

13.3. Rapid Enumeration and Selection Algorithms

If we are systematic and proceed in an orderly fashion from one rearrangement to the next, we can substantially reduce the time required to examine a series of rearrangements. Optimal algorithms for generating sequences of rearrangements are advanced by Walsh [1957]; Boothroyd [1967]; Plackett [1968]; Yangimoto and Okimnoto [1969]; Boulton [1974]; Hancock [1974]; Bitner, Ehrlich, and Rheingold [1976]; Akl [1981]; and Bissell [1986]. See, for example, the review by Wright [1984]. Recent minimal change algorithms include those of Berry [1982]; Lam and Sotchen [1982]; Nigam and Gupta [1984]; and Marsh [1987].

13.3.1. Matched Pairs

Sometimes we can reduce the number of computations that are required by taking advantage of the structure inherent in the way we label or identify individual permutations. In the case of paired comparisons, we readily enumerate each possible combination by running through the binary numbers from 0 to $2^n - 1$, letting the 0s and 1s in each number (obtained via successive right shifts, a single machine language instruction in most computers) correspond to positive and negative paired differences, respectively.

Censoring actually reduces the time required for enumeration. For if there are n_c censored pairs, then enumeration need only extend over the $2^{(n-n_c)}$ values that might be assumed by the uncensored pairs. In computing the GAMP test for paired comparisons, it is easy to see that

$$\Pr\{U' \geq U . \text{AND} . S' \geq S\} = \Pr\{U' \geq U\} * \Pr\{S' \geq S\}.$$

$$\Pr\{U' \geq U\} = \sum_{k=U}^{U+L} \binom{U + L}{k} \Big/ 2^{U+L}.$$

The remaining probability, $\Pr\{S' \geq S\}$, may be obtained by enumeration and inspection.

13.4. Focus on the Tails: Branch and Bound Algorithms

We can avoid examining all $N!$ rearrangements, if we focus on the tails, using the internal logic of the problem to deduce the number of rearrangements that yield values of the test statistic that are as extreme or more extreme than the original.

Green [1977] was the first to suggest a branch and bound method for use in two-sample tests and correlation. Our description of Green's method is based on [De Cani, 1979]:

In the two-sample comparison described in Section 3.2, suppose our test statistics, T, is $\sum_{l=1}^{m} x_{\pi(i)}$, and that the observed value is T_0. We seek $P(T \geq T_0)$, the probability under the null hypothesis that a random value of T equals or exceeds T_0.

Assume that the combined observations are arranged in descending order $X_{(1)} \geq X_{(2)} \geq \cdots \geq X_{(N)}$. To simplify the notation, let Z_i denote the ith order statistic $X_{(i)}$. If the labels (subscripts) on the X's really are irrelevant (as they would be under the null hypothesis) then T can be regarded as a random sample of m of the observations selected at random without replacement from the $\{Z_i\}$.

Suppose we have selected k such values, $Z_{I_1}, \ldots, Z_{I_k}, k < m$ The maximum attainable value of T is obtained by adding to $Z_{I_1} + \cdots + Z_{I_k}$ the $m - k$ largest of the $N - k$ remaining elements. Call this maximum $T(l_1, \ldots, l_k)$. Similarly, the minimum attainable value of T is obtained by adding to $Z_{I_1} + \cdots + Z_{I_k}$ the $m - k$ smallest of the $N - k$ remaining elements. Call this minimum $t(l_1, \ldots, l_k)$. Given $l_1, \ldots, l_k$, we can bound T:

$$t(l_1, \ldots, l_k) \leq T \leq T(l_1, \ldots, l_k).$$

There are $\binom{N - k}{m - k}$ sets of m elements of Z whose totals lie between the given bounds.

If $t(l_1, \ldots, l_k) \geq T_0$, then

$$P(T \geq T_0) \geq \binom{N - k}{m - k} \bigg/ \binom{N}{m}$$

If $T_0 > T(l_1, \ldots, l_k)$, then

$$P(T \geq T_0) \leq 1 - \binom{N - k}{m - k} \bigg/ \binom{N}{m}$$

If T_0 lies between the bounds, or if we require an improved bound on $P(T \geq T_0)$, then we can add a $k + 1$th element to the index set.

Our results apply equally to any test statistic of the form $\sum_{l=1}^{m} f[x_{\pi(i)}]$, where f is a monotone increasing function. Examples of such monotone functions include the logarithm (when applied to positive values), ranks, and any of the other robust transformations described in Chapter 9.

13.4.1. Contingency Tables

A large number of authors have joined in the search for a more rapid method for enumerating the tail probabilities for Fisher's exact test, including Leslie [1955]; Feldman and Kluger [1963]; Good [1976]; Gail and Mantel [1977]; Pagano and Halvorsen [1981]; and Patefield [1981]. See, for example, the review by Agresti [1993]. A quantum leap toward a more rapid method took place with the publication of the network approach of Mehta and Patel [1980]. Their approach is widely applicable, as we shall see below. It has three principal steps:

1. Representation of each contingency table as a path through a directed acyclic network with nodes and arcs
2. An algorithm with which to enumerate the paths in the tail of the distribution without tracing more than a small fraction of those paths
3. Determination of the smallest and largest path lengths at each node.

Only the last of these steps is application specific.
Network algorithms have been developed for all of the following:

$2 \times C$ contingency tables; [Mehta and Patel, 1980]
$R \times C$ contingency tables; [Mehta and Patel, 1983]
the common odds ratio in several 2×2 contingency tables [Mehta, Patel, and Gray, 1985]
logistic regression; [Hirji, Mehta, and Patel, 1987]
restricted clinical trials [Mehta, Patel, and Wei, 1988]
linear rank tests and the Mantel-Haenszel trend test [Mehta, Patel, and Senchaudhuri, 1988]

For simplicity, we focus in what follows on the $2 \times C$ contingency table.

13.4.1.1. Network Representation

Define the reference set Γ to be all possible $2 \times k$ contingency tables (see Chapter 6) with row marginals (m, n) and column marginals $(t_1, t_2, \ldots, t_k)$. Thus each table, $x \in \Gamma$, is of the form

$$
\begin{array}{ccccc}
x_1 & x_2 & \ldots & x_k & m \\
x_1' & x_2' & \ldots & x_k' & n \\
t_1 & t_2 & \ldots & t_k & N
\end{array}
$$

For each table $x \in \Gamma$, we may define a discrepancy measure

$$d(x) = \sum_{i=1}^{k} a_i(m_{i-1}, x_i)$$

and a probability

$$h(x) = C^{-1} \prod_{i=1}^{k} \lambda_i(m_{i-1}, x_i)$$

where the partial sum $m_j = \sum_{i=1}^{j} x_{i.}$, and the normalizing constant $C = \sum_{x \in \Gamma} \prod_{i=1}^{k} \lambda_i(m_{i-1}, x_i)$. Important special cases of $d(x)$ and $h(x)$ are

$$d(x) = \prod_{i=1}^{k} a_i x_i$$

for linear rank tests and

$$h(x) = \prod_{i=1}^{k} \binom{t_i}{x_i} \Big/ \binom{N}{m}$$

for unordered contingency tables.

As in Section 6.3, our object is to compute the one-sided significance level $p = \sum_R h(x)$, where R is the set on which $d(X) \geq d_0$.

First, we represent Γ as a directed acyclic network of nodes and arcs. Following Mehta and Patel [1983], the network is constructed recursively in $k + 1$ stages labelled $0, 1, 2, \ldots, k$. The nodes at the jth stage are ordered pairs (j, m_j) whose first element is j and whose second is the partial sum of the frequencies in the first j categories of the first row. If there is a total of 2 observations in the 1st category, then there will be three nodes at the first stage $(1, 0), (1, 1), (1, 2)$—corresponding to the three possible distributions of elements in this category.

Arcs emanate from the node (j, m_j); each arc is connected to exactly one successor node. Each path linking $(0, 0)$ with the terminal node (k, m) corresponds to a unique contingency table. For example, the path

$$(0, 0) \rightarrow (1, 0) \rightarrow (2, 2) \rightarrow (3, 4) \rightarrow (4, 4)$$

corresponds to the table

0	2	2	0	4
2	0	0	2	4
2	2	2	2	

The total number of paths in the network corresponds to the total number of tables. We could count the total number of tables by tracing each of the individual paths. But we can do better.

13.4.1.2. The Network Algorithm

Our goal in network terms is to quickly identify and sum all paths whose lengths do not exceed d·h: for the original unpermuted table. Let $\Gamma_j = \Gamma(j, m_j)$ denote the set of all paths from any node (j, m_j) to the terminal node (k, m). In other words. Γ_j represents all possible completions of those tables in Γ for which the sum of the first j cells of row 1 is m_j. Define the shortest path length

$$SP(j, m_j) = \min_{x \in \Gamma_j} \sum_{i=j+1}^{k} a_i(m_{i-1}, x_i)$$

and the longest path length

$$LP(j, m_j) = \max_{x \in \Gamma_j} \sum_{i=j+1}^{k} a_i(m_{i-1}, x_i).$$

Let $L(PAST)$ denote the length of a path from $(0,0)$ to (j, m_j). If this path is such that

$$L(\text{PAST}) + LP(j, m_j) \le d \cdot h,$$

then all similar subpaths from $(0,0)$ to (j, m_j) of equal or smaller length contribute to the p value. This number can be determined by induction—the details depend on the actual form of d and h, and thus we need not enumerate the tables explicitly. if this path is such that

$$L(\text{PAST}) + SP(j, m_j) \ge d \cdot h,$$

then we can ignore it and all similar paths of equal or greater length—again, without actually enumerating them.

If the path satisfies neither condition, then we extend it to a node at the $j + 1$th stage, compute the new shortest and longest path lengths and repeat the calculation.

The shortest and longest path lengths may be determined by dynamic programming in a single backward pass through the network. Dynamic programming is used by Mehta and Patel [1980] in their first seminal paper. Their original approach can be improved upon in three ways:

1) by taking advantage of the structure of the problem;
2) by a Monte Carlo, randomly selecting the successor node at each stage;
3) by a Monte Carlo utilizing importance sampling, that is, weighting the probabilities with which an available node is selected so as to reduce the variance of the resultant estimate of p.

The three approaches can be combined: A highly efficient two-pass algorithm for importance sampling using backward induction followed by forward induction was developed by Mehta, Patel, and Senchaudhuri [1988]. Their new algorithm guarantees that all rearrangements sampled will lie inside the critical region. A result of Joe [1988] also represents a substantial increase in computational efficiency.

13.5. Characteristic Functions

As the sample size increases, the number of possible rearrangements increases exponentially. For example, in the one-sample test of a location parameter based on n observations, there are 2^n possible rearrangements. When finding the permutation distribution of a statistic that is a linear combination of some function of the original observations, Pagano and Tritchler [1983] show we can reduce the computation time from $C_1 2^n$ to $C_2 n^c$ where c is, we hope, much less than n.

Their technique requires two steps: In the first, they determine the characteristic function of the permutation distribution through a set of difference equations. This step requires $2Qm(m + n)$ complex multiplications and additions to find the characteristic function at Q points. In the second, they use the basic theorem in Fourier series to invert the characteristic function and determine or approximate the permutation distribution at $U < Q$ different points. This step requires $2Q \log Q$ calculations. Q is normally chosen to be a power of 2 (e.g., 256 or 512) so that one can take advantage of a fast Fourier transform; the exact number will depend on the precision with which one wants to estimate the significance level.

This method is chiefly of historic interest; branch and bound algorithms offer greater computational efficiency, particularly when coupled with importance sampling. Vollset, Hirji, and Elashoff [1991] found that the fast Fourier transform method can result in considerable loss of numerical accuracy.

13.6. Asymptotic Approximations

13.6.1. A Central Limit Theorem

The fundamental asymptotic result for the permutation distribution of the two-sample test statistic for a location parameter was first stated by Madow [1948] and formalized by Hoeffding [1951, 1952] who demonstrates convergence of the distribution of the Studentized test statistic under the alternative as well as under the null hypothesis.

Let $T_n = T(X_{(1)}, \ldots, X_{(n)})$ be the test statistic and let μ_n and σ_n^2 be its first and second moments respectively. Then the permutation distribution F_n of

$$Z_n = \frac{T_n - \mu_n}{\sigma_n}$$ obtained by randomly rearranging the subscripts of the arguments of T_n converges to Φ, the Gaussian (normal) distribution function.

This result means that for sufficiently large samples, we can give our computers a rest, at least temporarily, and approximate the desired p-value with the aid of tables of the normal distribution. To use these tables, we need to know the first and second moments of the permutation distribution. Occasionally, with samples of moderate size, we may also need to know and use the third and higher moments in order to obtain an accurate approximation. Moments for the randomized block design are given by Pitman [1937] and Welch [1937], for the Latin Square by Welch [1937]; for the balanced incomplete block by Mitra [1961]; and for the completely randomized design by Robinson [1983], and Bradbury [1988].

Extensions to, and refinements of, Hoeffding's work are provided by Silvey [1954, 1956], Dwass [1955], Motoo [1957], Erdos and Renyi [1959], Hajek [1960, 1961], and Kolchin and Christyakov [1973]. Asymptotic results for rank tests are given in Jogdeo [1968] and Tardif [1981]. For further details of the practical application of asymptotic approximations to the analysis of complex experimental designs, see Lehmann [1986], Kempthorne, Zyskind, Addelman, Throckmorton, and White [1961], and Ogawa [1963].

13.6.2. Edgeworth Expansions

While the Gaussian distribution may provide a valid approximation to the *center* of the permutation distribution, it is the tails (and the *p*-values of the tails) with which we are primarily concerned. Edgeworth expansions give good approximations to the tails in many cases. Edgeworth expansions for the distribution function under both the alternative and the null hypothesis have been obtained by Albers, Bickel, and Van Zwet [1976], Bickel and Van Zwet [1978], Robinson [1978], and John and Robinson [1983].

Saddlepoint methods and large deviation results give still better approximations in the tails. Saddlepoint approximations for the one- and two-sample tests of location as suggested by Daniels [1955, 1958] are derived by Robinson [1982]. Saddlepoint approximations for use with general linear models for both the permutation distribution and the bootstrap are given by Booth and Butler [1990].

13.6.3. Generalized Correlation

Test statistics for location parameters are almost always linear or first-order functions of the observations. By contrast, test statistics for scale parameters, the chi-square statistic, and the Mantel-Valand statistic for generalized correlation are quadratic or second-order functions of the observations. Their limiting distributions are not Gaussian but chi-square or a Pearson type III distribution [Berry and Mielke, 1984, 1986, and Mielke and Berry, 1985]. Other asymptotic approximations for second-order statistics are given by Shapiro and Hubert [1979], O'Reilly and Mielke [1980], and Ascher and Bailar [1982].

13.7. Sample Size, Power, and Confidence Intervals

Suppose we are in the design stages of a study and we intend to use a permutation test for the analysis. How large should our sample sizes be? Our answer will depend on three things:

the alternative(s) of interest
the power desired at these alternatives
the significance level.

A not unrelated question arises if we conclude an analysis by accepting the null hypothesis. Does this mean the alternative is false or that we simply did not have a large enough sample to detect the deviation from the null hypothesis? Again, we must compute the power of the test for several alternatives before we are able to reach a decision.

We estimate the power by drawing a series of K (simulated) random samples from a distribution similar to that which would hold under the alternative. For each sample, we perform the permutation test at the stated significance level and record whether we accept or reject the null hypothesis. The proportion of rejections becomes our estimate of the power of the test.

When designing a study, I use $K = 100$ until I am ready to fine tune the sample size, when I switch to $K = 400$. I also study (estimate) the power for at least two distinct alternatives.

For example, when testing the hypothesis that the observations are normal with mean 0 against the alternative that they have a mean of at least 1, I will sample from alternatives with at least two different variances: say, one with variance equal to unity, and one with variance equal to 2, where 1 is my best guess of the unknown variance, and 2 is a worst-case possibility.

When doing an after-the-fact analysis of the power, I use estimates of the parameters based on the actual data. If the pooled sample variance is 1.5, then I use a best guess of 1.5 and a worst case of 3 or even 4. 1 may end by doing $8KN$ computations, where N is the average number of permutations I inspect each time I perform the test.

With such a large number of calculations, it is essential that I take advantage of one or more of the computational procedures described in Sections 2 through 6 of this chapter. Oden [1991] offers several recommendations. Gabriel and Hsu [1983] describe an application-specific method for reducing the number of computations required to estimate the power and determine the appropriate sample size.

13.8. Some Conclusions

In the Monte Carlo, we compute the test statistic for a sample of the possible rearrangements, and use the resultant sampling distribution and its percentiles in place of the actual permutation distribution and its percentiles. The drawback of this approach is that the resultant significance level p' may differ from the significance level p of a test based on the entire permutation distribution. p' is a consistant estimate of p with a standard deviation on the order of $Np(1 - p)$ where n is the number of rearrangements considered in the Monte Carlo.

In the original Monte Carlo, the rearrangements are drawn with equal probability. In a variant called *importance sampling*, the rearrangements are drawn with weights chosen so as to minimize the variance. In some instances, when combined with branch and bound techniques as in Mehta, Patel, and

Senchaudhuri [1988], importance sampling can markedly reduce the number of samples that are required. (See also Besag and Clifford [1989].)

A second drawback of the Monte Carlo is that selecting a random arrangement is itself a time-consuming operation that can take several multiples of the time required to compute the sample statistic. A current research focus is on rapid enumeration and selection algorithms that can provide a fast transition from one rearrangement to the next. To date, all solutions have been highly application-specific.

Branch and bound algorithms eliminate the need to evaluate each rearrangement individually. The network approach advanced by Mehta and Patel can cut computation time by several orders of magnitude. *STATXACT®*, a user-friendly program for IBM-PC compatible computers that uses the Mehta-Patel approach is available from Cytel Software, 137 Erie St, Cambridge MA 02139, 617/661-2011. *STATXACT* provides for two-sample comparisons, the logrank test for censored survival data, the Fisher exact test for 2×2 contingency tables, tests of $R \times C$ contingency tables, and tests for stratified contingency tables. Newer versions of the program offer importance sampling as an option.

Solutions through characteristic functions are seldom of practical interest. When subsamples are large—and it is the size of the subsample or block, not the sample as a whole, that is the determining factor—an asymptotic approximation should be considered. In my experience as an industrial statistician with the pharmaceutical and energy industries, the opportunity to take advantage of an asymptotic approximation seldom arises. In preclinical work, one seldom has enough observations. And in a clinical trial, though the sample size is large initially, one is usually forced to divide the sample again and again to correct for covariates. In practice, contingency tables always have one or two empty cells. The errors in significance level that can result from an inappropriate application of an asymptotic approximation are amply illustrated in Table 6.4.

If you are one of the favored few able to take advantage of an asymptotic approximation, you first will need to compute the mean and variance of the permutation distribution. In some cases, you will also need to calculate and use the third and fourth moments to increase the accuracy of the approximation. The calculations are different for each test, for details, consult the references in the corresponding sections of this text.

13.9. Questions

1. Most microcomputer-based random number generators use multiplicative congruence to produce a 16-bit unsigned integer between 0 and 2^{15}. Yet in the two-sample comparison, for example, we only use one of the 15 bits, the least significant bit, in selecting items for rearrangement. Could we use more of the bits? That is, are some or all of the bits independent of one another? Write algorithm(s) that take advantage of multiple bits.

2. Apply the Mehta and Patel approach to the following 3 × 2 contingency table:

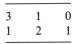

$$
\begin{array}{ccc}
3 & 1 & 0 \\
1 & 2 & 1
\end{array}
$$

Compute the marginals for this table. Draw a directed graph in which each node corresponds to a 3 × 2 table whose marginals are the same as those of the proceeding table. Choose a test statistic (see Section 6.3). Identify those nodes which give rise to a value of the test statistic less than that of the original table.

3. Suppose you are interested in the theoretical alternative

$$
\begin{array}{ccc}
4/6 & 1/6 & 1/6 \\
1/6 & 4/6 & 1/6
\end{array}
$$

How big a sample size would you need to insure that the probability of detecting this alternative was 80% at the 10% significance level? (Hint: use a six-sided die to simulate the drawing of samples.)

CHAPTER 14

Theory of Permutation Tests

In this chapter, we establish the underlying theory of permutation tests. The content is heavily mathematical, in contrast to previous chapters, and a knowledge of calculus is desirable.

14.1. Fundamental Concepts

In this section, we provide formal definitions for some of the concepts introduced in Chapter 2, including *distribution, power, exact, unbiased,* and the permutation test, itself.

14.1.1. Dollars and Decisions

A statistical problem is defined by three elements:

1) the class $F = (F_\theta, \theta \in \Omega)$ to which the probability distribution of the observations belongs; for example, we might specify that this distribution is unimodal, or symmetric, or normal;
2) the set D of possible decisions $\{d\}$ one can make on observing $X = (X_1, \ldots, X_n)$,
3) the loss $L(d, \theta)$, expressed in dollars, men's lives or some other quantifiable measure, that results when we make the decision d when θ is true.

A problem is a statistical one when the investigator is not in a position to say that X will take on exactly the value x, but only that X has some probability $P\{A\}$ of taking on values in the set A.

In this text, we've limited ourselves to two-sided decisions in which either we accept a hypothesis, H, and reject an alternative, K; or we reject the hypothesis, H, and accept the alternative, K.

One example is:

$$H: \theta \leq \theta_0$$

$$K: \theta > \theta_0.$$

In this example, we would probably follow up our decision to accept or reject with a confidence interval for the unknown parameter θ. This would take the form of an interval $(\theta_{min}, \theta_{max})$ and a statement to the effect that the probability that this interval covers the true parameter value is not less than $1 - \alpha$. This use of an interval can rescue us from the sometimes undesirable "all or nothing" dichotomy of hypothesis vs. alternative.

Another hypothesis/alternative pair which we considered in Section 3.6, under "testing for a dose response," is

$$H: \theta_1 = \cdots = \theta_J$$

$$K: \theta_1 < \cdots < \theta_J.$$

In this example, we might want to provide a confidence interval for $\max_j \theta_j - \min_j \theta_j$. Again, see Sections 3.2 and 7.4.

Typically, losses, L, depend on some function of the difference between the true (but unknown) value θ and our best guess θ^* of this value; $L(\theta, \theta^*) = |\theta - \theta^*|$ for example. In the first of the preceding examples, we might have

$$L(\theta, d) = \theta - \theta_0 \qquad \text{if } \theta \in K \text{ and } d = H,$$

$$L(\theta, d) = 10 \qquad \text{if } \theta \in H \text{ and } d = K,$$

$$L(\theta, d) = 0 \qquad \text{otherwise.}$$

Our objective is to come up with a decision rule, D, such that when we average out over *all* possible sets of observations X, we minimize the associated risk or expected loss,

$$R(\theta, D) = EL(\theta, D(X)).$$

Unfortunately, a testing procedure that is optimal for one value of the parameter, θ, might not be optimal for another. This situation is illustrated in Chapter 2, in Figure 2.4 with two decision curves that cross over each other. The risk, R, depends on θ and we don't know what the true value of θ is! How are we to choose the best decision?

This problem is complex with philosophical as well as mathematical overtones; we refer the interested reader to the discussions in the first chapter of Erich Lehmann's book, *Testing Statistical Hypotheses* [1986]. Our own solution in selecting an optimal test is to focus on the principle of unbiasedness discussed below in 14.1.3

14.1.2. Tests

A test, ϕ, is simply a decision rule that takes values between 0 and 1. When $\phi(x) = 1$, we reject the hypothesis and accept the alternative; when $\phi(x) = 0$, we accept the hypothesis and reject the alternative; and when $\phi(x) = p$, with $0 < p < 1$, we flip a coin that has been weighted so that the probability is p that it will come up heads, whence we reject the hypothesis, and $1 - p$ that it will come up tails, whence we accept the hypothesis.

An α-level permutation test consists of a vector of N observations z, a statistic $T[z]$, and an acceptance criterion $A: R \times R \to [0, 1]$, such that for all z, $\phi(z) = 1$ if and only if

$$W(z) = \sum_{\pi \in \Pi} A(T[z], T[\pi z]) \leq \alpha N!$$

where Π is the set of all possible rearrangements of the $n + m$ observations.

14.1.3. Distribution Functions, Power, Exact, and Unbiased Tests

The *distribution function* $F(x) = Pr\{X \leq x\}$; $F(x)$ is nondecreasing on the real line and $0 \leq F(x) \leq 1$. If F is continuous and differentiable, then it has a density $f(x)$ such that $\int_{-\infty}^{\infty} f(z)\,dz = F(x)$.

We define the *power* β_ϕ of a test ϕ based on a statistic X as the expectation of ϕ: $\beta_\phi(\theta) = E^\theta \phi(X) = \int_{-\infty}^{\infty} f\,dF_\theta$, where F_θ is the distribution of X. Note that β_ϕ is a function of the unknown parameter θ (and, possibly, of other, nuisance parameters as well). For the majority of the tests in this book, $\beta_\phi(\theta) = Pr\{\phi = 1|\theta\}$.

If θ satisfies the hypothesis, then $\beta_\phi(\theta)$ is the probability of making a Type I error if θ is true.

If θ satisfies the alternative, then $1 - \beta_\phi(\theta)$ is the probability of making a Type II error if θ is true.

A test, ϕ, is said to be *exact* with respect to a set ω of hypotheses if $E^H \phi = \alpha$, for all $H \in \omega$. A test is conservative under the same circumstances if $E^H \phi \leq \alpha$, for all $H \in \omega$. The use of an exact, and thus conservative, test guarantees that the Type I error will be held at or below a predetermined level.

A test, ϕ, is said to be *unbiased* and of level α providing that its power function β satisfies

$$\beta_\phi(\theta) \leq \alpha \text{ if } \theta \text{ satisfies the hypothesis}$$

$$\beta_\phi(\theta) \geq \alpha \text{ if } \theta \text{ satisfies one of the alternatives.}$$

That is, using an unbiased test, ϕ, you are more likely to reject a false hypothesis than a true one.

14.1.4. Exchangeable Observations

Suppose that $X_1, \ldots, X_n$ are distributed as $F(x)$, while $Y_1, \ldots, Y_n$ are distributed as $F(x - \delta)$, and that F has probability density f.

A sufficient condition for a permutation test to be exact is the *exchange-ability* of the observations [Lehmann, 1986, p. 231]. Let $S(z)$ be the set of points obtained from $z = (x_1, \ldots, x_m, y_1, \ldots, y_n)$ by permuting the coordinates of z in all $(n + m)!$ possible ways.

Theorem 1. *If F is the family of all $(n + m)$-dimensional distributions with probability densities, f, that are integrable and symmetric in their arguments, and we wish to test alternatives of the form $f(x_1, \ldots, x_m, y_1 - \delta, \ldots, y_n - \delta)$ against the hypothesis that $\delta = 0$, a test ϕ is unbiased for all $f \in F$ if and only if $\sum_{z' \in S(z)} \phi(z') = \alpha(n + m)!$ a.e.*

The proof of this result relies on the fact that the set of order statistics constitute a complete sufficient statistic for F. See, for example, Lehmann [1986, pp. 45–6, 143–4, 231]. Also see problem 2 in this Chapter. For more on exchangeability, see Koch [1982], and Romano [1990].

14.2. Maximizing the Power

In this section, we set about deriving the most powerful unbiased test for the two-sample testing problem. We will show that the two-sample test for a location parameter is unbiased against stochastically increasing alternatives. We define the likelihood ratio and restate, without proof, the fundamental theorem of Neyman and Pearson. We apply this theorem to show that the two-sample permutation test based on the sum of the observations is uniformly most powerful among unbiased tests against normal alternatives. Finally, we establish the intimate interdependence of confidence intervals and hypothesis tests. We follow closely the derivations provided in Lehmann [1986].

14.2.1. Uniformly Most Powerful Unbiased Tests

A family of cumulative distribution functions is said to be *stochastically increasing* if the distributions are distinct and if $\theta < \theta'$ implies $F_\theta(x) \geq F_{\theta'}(x)$ for all x. One example is the location parameter family for which $F_\theta(x) = F(x - \theta)$. If X and X' have distributions F_θ and F'_θ, then $P\{X > x\} \leq P(X' > x)$, that is, X' tends to have larger values than X. Formally, we say that X' is *stochastically larger* than X.

Lemma 1. *$F_1(x) \leq F_0(x)$ for all x only if there exist two nondecreasing functions f_0 and f_1 and a random variable V such that $f_0 \leq f_1$ for all v and the distributions of f_0 and f_1 are F_0 and F_1 respectively.*

Proof. Set $f_i(y) = \inf\{x : F_i(x - 0) \leq y \leq F_i(x)\}$, $i = 0, 1$. These functions are nondecreasing and for $f_i = f$, $F_i = F$ satisfy $f[F(x)] \leq x$ and $F[f(y)] \geq y$ for all x and y. Thus, $y \leq F(x_0)$ implies $f(y) \leq f[F(x_0)] \leq x_0$ and $f(y) \leq x_0$ implies $F[f(y)] \leq F(x_0)$ implies $y \leq F(x_0)$.

Let V be uniformly distributed on $(0, 1)$. Then $P\{f_i(V) \leq x\} = P\{V \leq F_i(x)\}$ $= F_i(x)$ which completes the proof. $\square$

We can apply this result immediately:

Lemma 2. *Let* $X_1, \ldots, X_m; Y_1, \ldots, Y_n$ *be samples from continuous distributions* F, G, *and let* $\phi[X_1, \ldots, X_m; Y_1, \ldots, Y_n]$ *be a test such that* a) *whenever* $F = G$, *its expectation is* α; *and* b) $y_i \leq y_i'$ *for* $1 = 1, \ldots, n$ *implies* $\phi[x_1, \ldots, x_m;$ $y_1, \ldots, y_n] \leq \phi[x_1, \ldots, x_m; y_1', \ldots, y_n']$. *Then the expectation of* ϕ *is greater than or equal to* α *for all pairs of distributions for which* Y *is stochastically larger than* X.

Proof. From our first lemma, we know there exist functions, f and g, and independent random variables, $V_1, \ldots, V_{m+n}$, such that the distributions of $f(V_i)$ and $g(V_i)$ are F and G respectively and $f(z) \leq g(z)$ for all z.

$$E\phi[f(V_1), \ldots, f(V_m); f(V_1), \ldots, f(V_n)] = \alpha$$

and

$$E\phi[f(V_1), \ldots, f(V_m); g(V_1), \ldots, g(V_n)] = \beta.$$

From condition b) of the lemma, we see that $\beta > \alpha$ as was to be proved. $\square$

We are now in a position to state the principal result of this section:

Theorem 2 (Unbiased). *Let* $X_1, \ldots, X_m; Y_1, \ldots, Y_n$ *be samples from continuous distributions* F, G. *Let* $\beta(F, G)$ *be the expectation of the critical function* ϕ *defined in* (14.1); *that is,* $\phi[X_1, \ldots, X_m; Y_1, \ldots, Y_n] = 1$ *only if* $\sum Y_j$ *is greater than the equivalent sum in* α *of the* $\binom{n + m}{n}$ *possible rearrangements. Then* $\beta(F, F) = \alpha$ *and* $\beta(F, G) \geq \alpha$ *for all pairs of distributions for which* Y *is stochastically larger than* X; $\beta(F, G) \leq \alpha$ *if* X *is stochastically larger than* Y.

Proof. $\beta(F, F) = \alpha$, follows from Theorem 1 and the definition of ϕ. We can apply our lemmas and establish that the two-sample permutation test is unbiased if we can show that $y_j \leq y_j'$ for $j = 1, \ldots, n$ implies

$$\phi[x_1, \ldots, x_m; y_1, \ldots, y_n] \leq \phi[x_1, \ldots, x_m; y_1', \ldots, y_n'].$$

$\phi = 1$ if sufficiently many of the differences

$$d(\pi) = \sum_{i=m+1}^{m+n} z_i - \sum_{i=m+1}^{m+n} z_{j_i}$$

are positive. For a particular permutation $\pi = (j_1, \ldots, j_{m+n})$,

$$d(\pi) = \sum_{i=1}^{p} z_{s_i} - \sum_{i=m+1}^{p} z_{r_i}$$

where $r_1 < \cdots < r_p$ denote those of the integers $j_{m+1}, \ldots, j_{m+n}$ that are less than or equal to m, and $s_1 < \cdots < s_p$ denote those of the integers $m + 1, \ldots,$ $m + n$ that are not included in the set $(j_{m+1}, \ldots, j_{m+n})$.

If $\sum z_{s_i} - \sum z_{r_i}$ is positive and $y_i \le y'_i$, that is $z_i \le z'_i$ for $i = m + 1, \ldots,$ $m + n$, then the difference $\sum z'_{s_i} - \sum z_{r_i}$ is also positive; so that $\phi(z') \ge \phi(z)$. But then we may apply the lemmas to obtain the desired result. The proof is similar for the case in which X is stochastically larger than Y. $\square$

14.2.2. The Fundamental Lemma

In Section 10.4, we showed that if the variables take only a countable number of values, then the most powerful test of a simple hypothesis P_0 against a simple alternative P_1 rejects the hypothesis in favor of the alternative only for those values of x with the largest values of the likelihood ratio

$$r(x) = \frac{p_1(x)}{p_0(x)}.$$

We can extend this result to continuous distribution functions with the aid of the fundamental lemma of Neyman and Pearson:

Theorem 3. *Let P_0 and P_1 be probability distributions possessing densities p_0 and p_1 respectively.*
   a) *There exists a test ϕ and a constant k such that*

$$E_0\phi(X) = \alpha$$

and

$$\phi(x) = \begin{array}{ll} 1 & when \quad p_1(x) > kp_0(x) \\ 0 & when \quad p_1(x) > kp_0(x). \end{array}$$

   b) *A test that satisfies these conditions for some k is most powerful for testing p_1 against p_0 at level α.*
   c) *If ϕ is most powerful for testing p_1 against p_0 at level α, then for some k it satisfies these conditions (except on a set that is assigned probability zero by both distributions and unless there exists a test at a smaller significance level whose power is 1).*

A proof of this seminal lemma is given in Lehmann [1986, p. 74].

Let z denote a vector of $n + m$ observations, and let $S(z)$ be the set of points obtained from z by permuting the coordinates z_i $(i = 1, \ldots, n + m)$ in all $(n + m)!$ possible ways.

Among all the unbiased tests of the null hypothesis that two sets of observations come from the same distribution, which satisfy the permutation condition

$$\sum_{z' \in S(z)} \phi(z') = \alpha(n + m)!,$$

which is the most powerful?

Let $t = T(z)$ denote the corresponding set of order statistics $(z_{(1)} < z_{(2)} < \cdots < z_{(n+m)})$. Lehmann [1986, p. 232] showed that the problem of maximizing the power of a test ϕ subject to the permutation condition against an alternative with arbitrary fixed density, h, reduces to maximizing

$$\sum_{z \in S(t)} \phi(z) \frac{h(z)}{\sum\limits_{z' \in S(t)} h(z')}.$$

By the fundamental lemma of Neyman and Pearson, this expression is maximized by rejecting the hypothesis and setting $\phi(z) = 1$ for those points z of $S(t)$ for which the ratio

$$h(z) \bigg/ \sum_{z' \in S(t)} h(z') \tag{14.1}$$

is largest. The most powerful unbiased α-level test is given by rejecting when $h(z) > C[T(z), \alpha]$ and accepting when $h(z) < C[T(z), \alpha]$. To achieve α exactly, it may also be necessary to use a chance device and to reject with some probability, γ, if $h(z) = C[T(z), \alpha]$.

To carry out this test, we order the permutations according to the values of the density h. We reject the hypothesis for the k largest of the values, where

$$k \le \alpha(n + m)! \le k + 1.$$

The critical value C depends on the sample through its order statistics T and on the density h. Thus different distributions for X will give rise to different optimal tests.

14.2.3. Samples from a Normal Distribution

In what follows, we consider three applications of the likelihood ratio: testing for the equality of the location parameters in two populations, testing for the equality of the variances, and testing for bivariate correlation.

Suppose that $Z_1, \ldots, Z_m$ and $Z_{m+1}, \ldots, Z_{n+m}$ are independent random samples from normal populations $N(\eta, \sigma^2)$ and $N(\eta + \delta, \sigma^2)$. Then

$$h(z) = (2\pi\sigma)^{-N/2} \exp\left[-\frac{1}{2\sigma^2} \left(\sum_{j=1}^{m} (z_j - \eta)^2 + \sum_{j=m+1}^{n+m} (z_j - \eta - \delta)^2 \right) \right].$$

$$= (2\pi\sigma)^{-N/2} \exp\left[-\frac{1}{2\sigma^2} \left(\sum_{j=1}^{n+m} (z_j - \eta)^2 - 2\delta \sum_{j=m+1}^{n+m} (z_j - \eta) + n\delta^2 \right) \right].$$

Before substituting this expression in our formula, 14.1, we may eliminate all factors which remain constant under permutations of the subscripts. These include $(2\pi\sigma)^{-(n+m)/2}$, $n\delta(\delta + \eta)$, and $\sum_{j=1}^{n+m}(z_j - \eta)^2$. The resulting test rejects when $\exp\left[\delta \sum_{j=m+1}^{n+m} z_j\right] > C[T(z), \alpha]$ or, equivalently, when the sum of the observations in the treated sample $\sum z_j$ is large. This sum can take at most $(n + m)!$ possible values and our rejection region consists of the $\alpha(n + m)!$ largest.

This permutation test is the same whatever the unknown values of η and σ and thus is uniformly most powerful against normally-distributed alternatives among all unbiased tests of the hypothesis that the two samples come from the same population.

14.2.4. Testing the Equality of Variances

As a second and elementary illustration of the likelihood ratio approach, suppose we are given that $z_1, \ldots, z_n$ are independent and identically normally distributed with mean 0 and variance σ^2, $N(0, \sigma^2)$, and that $z_{n+1}, \ldots, z_{m+n}$ are independent and identically normally distributed with mean 0 and variance τ^2, $N(0, \tau^2)$. We wish to test the hypothesis that $\sigma^2 = \tau^2$ against the alternative that $\sigma^2 < \tau^2$.

Let $\theta = \tau^2/\sigma^2$ and note that hypothesis and alternative may be rewritten as $H: \theta = 1$ vs $K: \theta > 1$.

$$\text{Then } h(z) = (2\pi)^{-(n+m)/2}\sigma^{-m}\tau^{-n}\exp\left[-\frac{1}{2\sigma^2}\sum_{j=1}^{n} z_j^2 + \frac{1}{2\tau^2}\sum_{j=m+1}^{n+m} z_j^2\right]$$

$$= (2\pi\sigma)^{-(n+m)/2}\theta^{-n/2}\exp\left[-\frac{1}{2\tau^2}\left(\theta\sum_{j=1}^{n} z_j^2 + \sum_{j=m+1}^{n+m} z_j^2\right)\right]$$

$$= (2\pi\sigma)^{-(n+m)/2}\theta^{-n/2}\exp\left[-\frac{1}{2\tau^2}\left((\theta - 1)\sum_{j=1}^{n} z_j^2 + \sum_{j=1}^{n+m} z_j^2\right)\right].$$

Eliminating terms that are invariant under permutations of the combined sample, such as the sum of the squares of all $n + m$ observations, we are left with the expression

$$\exp\left[-\frac{1}{2\tau^2}(\theta - 1)\sum_{j=1}^{n} z_j^2\right].$$

Our test statistic is the sum of the squares of the observations in the first sample.

14.2.5. Testing for Bivariate Correlation

Suppose we have made N simultaneous observations on the pair of variables X, Y and wish to test the alternative of positive dependence of Y on X against the null hypothesis of independence. In formal terms, if Y_x is the random variable whose distribution is the conditional distribution of Y given that $X = x$, we want to test the null hypothesis that Y_x has the same distribution for all x, against the alternative that if $x' > x$, then $Y_{x'}$ is likely to be larger than Y_x.

To find a most powerful test of this hypothesis that is unbiased against alternatives with probability density $h(z)$, we need to maximize the expression

$$\sum_{z \in S(t)} \phi(z) \frac{h(z)}{\sum_{z' \in S(t)} h(z')}.$$

For bivariate normal alternatives,

$$h(z) = (2\pi\sigma\tau\sqrt{1 - \rho^2})^{-n} \exp\left[-\frac{A}{2(1 - \rho^2)}\right]$$

where $A = \frac{1}{2\sigma^2} \sum_{j=1}^{n} (x_j - \eta)^2 + \frac{2\rho}{\sigma\tau} \sum_{j=1}^{n} (x_j - \eta)(y_j - v) + \frac{1}{2\tau^2} \sum_{j=1}^{n} (y_j - v)^2$.

Many of the sums that occur in this expression are invariant under permutations of the subscripts j. These include the four sums $\sum x_j$, $\sum y_j$, $\sum x_j^2$, $\sum y_j^2$. Eliminating all these invariant terms leaves us with the test statistic $r = \sum x_j y_{\pi(j)}$.

We evaluate this statistic both for the original data and for all $n!$ permutations of the subscripts of the y's, keeping the subscripts on the x's fixed. We reject the null hypothesis in favor of the alternative of positive dependence only if the original value of the test statistic exceeds all but $\alpha\%$ of the values for the rearrangements.

Reordering the x's so that $x_{(1)} \leq x_{(2)} \leq \ldots \leq x_{(n)}$, we see that this test is equivalent to using Pitman correlation (Section 3.5) to test the hypothesis of the randomness of the y's against the alternative of an upward trend.

14.3. Confidence Intervals

Let $x = \{X_1, X_2, \ldots, X_n\}$ be an exchangeable sample from a distribution, F_θ, which depends upon a parameter, $\theta \in \Omega$. A family of subsets, $S(x)$, of the parameter space Ω is said to be a family of confidence sets for θ at level $1 - \alpha$ if

$$P_\theta\{\theta' \in S(X)\} \geq 1 - \alpha \qquad \text{for all } \theta \in H(\theta').$$

The family is said to be unbiased if

$$P_\theta\{\theta' \in S(X)\} \leq 1 - \alpha \qquad \text{for all } \theta \in \Omega - H(\theta').$$

The construction of a confidence set from a family of acceptance regions is described in Chapter 3. The following theorem shows us this construction can proceed in either direction.

Theorem 4.1. *For each $\theta' \in \Omega$, let $A(\theta')$ be the acceptance region of the level-α test for $H(\theta')$: $\theta = \theta'$, and for each sample point, x, let $S(x)$ denote the set of parameter values $\{\theta: x \in A(\theta), \theta \in \Omega\}$. Then $S(x)$ is a family of confidence sets for θ at confidence level $1 - \alpha$.*

4.2. If for all θ', $A(\theta')$ is UMPU for testing $H(\theta')$ at level α against the alternatives $K(\theta')$, then for each θ' in Ω, $S(X)$ minimizes the probability

$$P_\theta\{\theta' \in S(X)\} \qquad \text{for all } \theta \in K(\theta')$$

among all unbiased level $1 - \alpha$ family of confidence sets for θ.

Proof 4.1. By definition, $\theta \in S(x)$ if and only if $x \in A(\theta)$, hence $P_\theta\{\theta \in S(X)\} = P_\theta\{X \in A(\theta)\} \geq 1 - \alpha$.

Proof 4.2. If $S^*(x)$ is any other family of unbiased confidence sets at level $1 - \alpha$ and if $A^*(\theta) = \{x: \theta \in S^*(x)\}$, then

$$P_\theta\{X \in A^*(\theta')\} = P_\theta\{\theta' \in S^*(x)\} \geq 1 - \alpha \qquad \text{for all } \theta \in H(\theta'),$$

and

$$P_\theta\{X \in A^*(\theta')\} = P_\theta\{\theta' \in S^*(X)\} \leq 1 - \alpha \qquad \text{for all } \theta \in \Omega - H(\theta'),$$

so that $A^*(q')$ is the acceptance region of a level-α unbiased test of $H(\theta')$. Since A is $UMPU$,

$$P_\theta\{X \in A^*(\theta')\} \geq P_\theta\{X \in A(\theta')\} \qquad \text{for all } \theta \in \Omega - H(\theta'),$$

hence $P_\theta\{\theta' \in S^*(x)\} \geq P_\theta\{\theta' \in S(x)\}$ for all $\theta \in \Omega - H(\theta')$, as was to be proved. $\square$

14.4. Asymptotic Behavior

A major reason for the popularity of the permutation tests is that with very large samples their power is almost indistinguishable from that of the most powerful parametric tests. To establish this result, we need to know something about the distribution of the permutation statistics as the sample size increases without limit. Two sets of results are available to us. The first, due to Wald and Wolfowitz [1947] and Hoeffding [1953] provides us with conditions under which the limiting distribution is normal under the null hypothesis; the second, due to Albers, Bickel, and Van Zwet [1976] and Bickel and Van Zwet [1978] provides conditions under which this distribution is normal for near alternatives.

14.4.1. A Theorem on Linear Forms

Let $S_N = (s_{N1}, s_{N2}, \ldots, s_{NN})$ and $U_N = (u_{N1}, u_{N2}, \ldots, u_{NN})$ be sequences of real numbers and let $s_{N.} = \sum s_{Nj}/N$; $u_{N.} = \sum u_{Nj}/N$.

The sequences S_N satisfy the condition W, if for all integers $r > 2$,

$$W(S_N, r) = \frac{|\sum (s_{Nj} - s_{N.})^r|}{\sum [(s_{Nj} - s_{N.})^2]^{r/2}} \text{ is bounded above for all } n.$$

The sequences S_N, U_N jointly satisfy the condition H_1, if for all integers $r > 2$,

$$\lim_N N^{r/2 - 1} W(S_N, r) W(U_N, r) = 0$$

The sequences S_N, U_N jointly satisfy the condition H_2, if for all integers $r > 2$,

$$\lim_N N \frac{\max_j (s_{Nj} - s_{N.})^r}{\sum (s_{Nj} - s_{N.})^r} \frac{\max_j (u_{Nj} - u_{N.})^r}{\sum (u_{Nj} - u_{N.})^r}$$

For any value of N let $X = (x_1, x_2, \ldots, x_N)$ be a chance variable whose possible values correspond to the $N!$ permutations of the sequence $A_N = (a_1, a_2, \ldots, a_N)$. Let each permutation of A_N have the same probability $1/N!$ and let $E(Y)$ and $SD(Y)$ denote the expectation and standard deviation of the variable Y.

Theorem 5. *Let the sequences* $A_N = (a_1, a_2, \ldots, a_N)$ *and* $D_N = (d_1, d_2, \ldots, d_N)$ *for* $N = 1, 2, \ldots$, *satisfy any of the three conditions* W, H_1, *and* H_2. *Let the chance variable* L_N *be defined as* $L_N = \sum d_i x_i$. *Then as* $N \to \infty$,

$$Pr\{L_N - E(L_N) < t SD(L_N)\} \to \frac{1}{\sqrt{2\pi}} \int_{-\infty}^{t} e^{-x^2/2} \, dx.$$

A proof of this result for condition W is given in Wald and Wolfowitz [1944]. The proof for conditions H_1 and H_2 is given in Hoeffding [1953].

This theorem applies to the majority of the tests we have already considered, including:

1) Pitman's correlation $\sum d_i a_i$;
2) the two-sample test with observations $a_1, \ldots, a_{m+n}$; and d_i equal to one if $i = 1, \ldots, m$ and zero otherwise,
3) Hotelling's T with $\{a_{1j}\}$ and $\{a_{2j}\}$ the observations—both sequences must separately satisfy the conditions of the theorem, and $d_i = 1/m$ for $i = 1$, $\ldots, m$; $d_i = -1/n$ for $i = m + 1, \ldots, m + n$.

14.4.2. Asymptotic Efficiency

In this section, we provide asymptotic expansions to order N^{-1} for the power of the one- and two-sample permutation tests and compare them with the asymptotic expansions for the most powerful parametric unbiased tests. The general expansion takes the form

$$b_N = c_0 + c_1 N^{-1/2} + c_{2,N} N^{-1} + o(N^{-1}),$$

where the coefficients depend on the form of the distribution, the significance level, and the alternative—but in both the one- and two-sample cases, the expansions for the permutation test and the t-test coincide for all terms through N^{-1}. The underlying assumptions are: 1) the observations are independent; 2) within each sample they are identically distributed; and 3) the two populations differ at most by a shift, $G(x) = F(x - \delta)$ where $\delta \geq 0$. $\beta(p, F, \delta)$ and $\beta(t, F, \delta)$ are the power functions of the permutation test and the parametric t-test, respectfully (see Section 2.3). The theorem's other restrictions are technical in nature and provide few or no limitations in practice; e.g., the significance level must lie between 0 and 1 and the distribution must have absolute moments of at least 9th order. We state the theorem for the one-sample case only.

Theorem 6. *Suppose the distribution F is continuous and that positive numbers C, D, and $r > 8$ exist such that $\int |x|^r \, dF[x] \leq C$ and $0 \leq \delta \leq DN^{-1/2}$, then if α is neither 0 nor 1, there exists a $B > 0$ depending on C and D, and a $b > 0$ depending only on r such that $|\beta(p, F, \delta) - \beta(t, F, \delta)| \leq BN^{-1/b}$.*

Proof of this result and details of the expansion are given in Bickel and Van Zwet [1976]. The practical implication is that for large samples the permutation test and the parametric t-test make equally efficient use of the data.

Robinson [1989] finds approximately the same coverage probabilities for three sets of confidence intervals for the slope of a simple linear regression based, respectively, on: 1) the standardized bootstrap; 2) parametric theory; and 3) a permutation procedure. Under the standard parametric assumptions, the coverage probabilities differ by $o(n^{-1})$, and the intervals themselves differ by $O(n^{-1})$ on a set of probability $1 - O(n^{-1})$.

14.4.3. Exchangeability

The requirement that the observations be exchangeable can be relaxed at least asymptotically for some one-sample and two-sample tests. Let $X_1, \ldots, X_n$ be a sample from a distribution F that may or may not be symmetric. Let $R_n(x, \Pi_n)$ be the permutation distribution of the statistic $T_n(X_1, \ldots, X_n)$ and let r_n denote the critical value of the associated permutation test; let $J_n(x, F)$ be the unconditional distribution of this same statistic under F; and let Φ denote the standard normal distribution function.

Theorem 7 *If F has mean 0 and finite variance $\sigma^2 > 0$, and $T_n = n^{1/2} \bar{X}$ then as $n \to \infty$,*

$$\sup_x |R_n(x, \Pi_n) - J_n(x, F)| \to 0 \text{ with probability 1,}$$

and $\sup_x |R_n(x, \Pi_n) - \Phi(x/\sigma)| \to 0$ *with probability 1. Thus* $r_n \to \sigma z_a$, *with probability 1 and* $E_F[\phi(R_n)] \to \alpha$.

A proof of this one-sample result is given in Romano [1990]; a similar one-sample result holds for a permutation test of the median subject to some mild continuity restrictions in the neighborhood of the median.

The two-sample case is quite different. Romano [1990] shows that if F_X and F_Y have common mean μ and finite variances σ_X^2 and σ_Y^2, respectively, $T_{m,n} = n^{1/2}(\overline{X} - \overline{Y})$, and $m/n \to \lambda$ as $n \to \infty$, the unconditional distribution of $T_{m,n}$ is asymptotically Gaussian with mean 0 and variance $\sigma_X^2 + (1 - \lambda)\sigma_Y^2/\lambda$ while the permutation distribution of $T_{m,n}$ is asymptotically Gaussian with mean 0 and variance $\sigma_Y^2 + (1 - \lambda)\sigma_X^2/\lambda$. Thus, the two asymptotic distributions are the same only if either a) the variances of the two populations are the same, or b) the sizes of the two samples are equal (whence $\lambda = 1$).

Romano also shows that whatever the sample sizes, a permutation test for the difference of the medians of two populations will not be exact, even asymptotically (except in rare circumstances) unless the underlying distributions are the same.

14.5. Questions

1. **Unbiased.** The test $\phi \equiv \alpha$ is a great timesaver; you don't have to analyze the data; you don't even have to gather data! All you have to do is flip a coin.
   a) Prove that this test is unbiased.
   b) Prove that a biased test cannot be uniformly most powerful.

2. **Sufficiency.** A statistic, T, is said to be sufficient for a family of distributions $P = \{P_\theta, \theta \in \Omega\}$ (or sufficient for θ) if the conditional probability of an event given $T = t$ is independent of θ.
   a) Let $x_1, \ldots, x_n$ be independent, identically distributed observations from a continuous distribution F_θ. Show that the set of order statistics $T = \{x_{(1)} < \cdots < x_{(1)}\}$ is sufficient for θ.
   b) Let $x_1, \ldots, x_n$ be a sample from a uniform distribution $U(0, \theta)$, with density $h(x) = 1/\theta$, that is, $P(x \leq u) = u/\theta$ for $0 \leq u \leq \theta$. Show that $T = \max(x_1, \ldots, x_n)$ is sufficient for θ.
   c) Let $x_1, \ldots, x_n$ be a sample from the exponential distribution with density $\frac{1}{b} e^{-(x-a)/b}$, $b > 0$. Show that the pair $\{\min(x_1, \ldots, x_n), \sum x_i\}$ is sufficient for a, b.

3. **Likelihood ratio.**
   a) Suppose that $\{X_i, i = 1, \ldots, n\}$ is $N(\mu, \sigma^2)$ and $\{Y_i, i = 1, \ldots, m\}$ is $N(\mu, \tau^2)$. Derive the most powerful unbiased permutation test for testing $H: \tau^2/\sigma^2 = 1$ against $not H: \tau^2/\sigma^2 = 2$.
   b) The times between successive decays of a radioactive isotope are said to follow the exponential distribution, that is, the probability that an atom will not decay until after an interval of length t is $1 - \exp[-t/\lambda]$. (A similar formula provides

a first-order approximation to the time, t, you will spend waiting for the next bus.) Suppose you had two potentially different isotopes with parameters λ_1 and λ_2 respectively. Derive a *UMPU* permutation test for testing $H: \lambda_1 = \lambda_2$, against $not H: \lambda_1 > \lambda_2$.

c) More generally, suppose that an item is reliable for a fixed period, b, after which its reliability decays at a constant rate λ. Then its lifetime has the exponential density $\lambda^{-1} \exp[x - b]/\lambda$. What statistic would you use for testing that $H: \lambda_1 = \lambda_2$, against not $H: \lambda_1 > \lambda_2$? Is your answer the same as in 2b)? Why not? (Hint: Look for sufficient statistics. Note that the problem remains invariant under an arbitrary scale transformation applied to both sets of data. And see Section 3.4).

Bibliography

For your convenience, this bibliography is divided into four parts.

The first, main bibliography, is of the research literature on permutation tests from the introduction of this straightforward approach to hypothesis testing by E.J.G. Pitman and R.A. Fisher in the mid 1930s to the present date. Each citation in this section is indexed in accordance with the nature of its contribution—concept, (univariate) test, algorithm, multivariate (test) and so forth.

A second, supporting bibliography, consists of articles we have cited in the text but which are not articles on permutation per se.

Since so much of today's research on permutation tests focuses on methods of rapid computation, we include a third, separate bibliography on computational methods.

A final and fourth bibliography consists of those few papers which we consider seminal both to an understanding of permutation tests and to the development of the subsequent vast wealth of articles on the topic. We hope every reader will select readings from this latter bibliography along with articles which are specific to her own interests.

In forming these bibliographies, we restricted ourselves to material on permutations and permutation tests which was directly related to hypothesis testing and estimation. Although, strictly speaking, every rank test is a permutation test, we did not include articles on rank tests in the bibliography unless, as is the case with some seminal work on multivariate analysis, the material is essential to an understanding of all permutation tests. Conference proceedings are excluded, the expected exception being a seminal paper by John Tukey which is available in no other form.

We have tried to be comprehensive, yet selective, and have personally read all but three of the articles in the bibliography. We hope you will find this bibliography of value in your work. We would appreciate your drawing to our attention articles on the theory and application of permutation tests which we may have excluded inadvertently.

Randomization

1. Adamson P; I Hajimohamadenza, M Brammer and IC Campbell. Intrasynato-somal free calcium concentration is increased by phobol esters via a 1,4-dihydro-pyridine-sensitive (I-type) CA2+. *European J Pharmacy*; 1989; 162: 59–66. application.
2. Adderley EE. Nonparametric methods of analysis applied to large-scale seeding experiments. *J Meteor*; 1961; 18: 692–694. application.
3. Agresti A. *Categorical Data Analysis*. New York: John Wiley & Sons; 1990. xtab.
4. Agresti A. A survey of exact inference for contingency tables. *Statistical Science*; 1992; 7: 131–177. xtab/concept/algorithm/review.
5. Agresti A; JB Lang and C Mehta. Some empirical comparisons of exact, modified exact, and higher-order asymptotic tests of independence for ordered categorical variables. *Commun Statist—Simul*; 1993; 22: 1–18. cross-tab/Monte Carlo.
6. Agresti A; CR Mehta and NR Patel. Exact inference for contingency tables with ordered categories. *J Am Stat Assoc*, 1990; 85: 453–458.
7. Agresti A; D Wackerly and JM Boyett. Exact conditional tests for cross-classifi-cations: approximations of attained significance levels. *Psychometrika*; 1979; 44: 75–83. tests.
8. Agresti A; D Wackerly. Some exact conditional tests of independence for $R \times C$ cross-classification tables. *Psychometrika*; 1977; 42: 111–126. algorithm/independence.
9. Albers W; PJ Bickel and WR Van Zwet. Asymptotic expansions for the power of distribution-free tests in the one-sample problem. *Annal Stat*; 1976; 4: 108–156. power/asymptotic.
10. Albert A; JP Chapelle, C Huesghem, GE Kulbertus and EK Harris. *Advanced Interpretation of Clinical Laboratory Data*. C Huesghem, A Albert and ES Benson. New York: Marcel Dekker; 1982. application.
11. Alderson MR; R Nayak. A study of space-time clustering in Hodgkin's disease in the Manchester Region. *Brit J Prev Soc Med*; 1971; 25: 168–73. cluster/application.
12. Andersen PK; O Borgan, R Gill and N Keiding. Linear nonparametric tests for

comparison of counting processes with applications to censored survival data. *Int Statist Rev*; 1982; 50: 219–58.
censor/survival.

13. Andres AM. A review of classic non-asymptotic methods for comparing two proportions by means of independent samples. *Commun Statist—Simul*; 1991; 20: 551–583.
xtab/power.

14. Armitage P. *Statistical Methods in Medical Research*. New York: John Wiley & Sons; 1971.
Fisher's exact.

15. Arnold HJ. Permutation support for multivariate techniques. *Biometrika*; 1964; 51: 65–70.
multivariate.

16. Ascher S; J Bailar. Moments of the Mantel-Valand procedure. *J Statist Comput Simul*; 1982; 14: 101–111.
asymptotic.

17. Baglivo J; D Olivier, and M Pagano. Methods for the analysis of contingency tables with large and small cell counts. *J Am Statist Assoc*, 1988; 83: 1006–1013.
algorithm/xtab.

18. Bahadur, RR; M Raghavachari. Some asymptotic properties of likelihood ratios on general sample spaces. in E LeCam and L Neyman Eds. Sixth Berkeley Symposium of Mathematical Statistics and Probability. Berkeley CA: University of California Press; 1970: 129–152.
theory.

19. Bailer, A John. Testing variance equality with randomization tests. *J Statist Comput Simul*; 1989; 31: 1–8.
tests.

20. Baker FB; RO Collier. Some empirical results on variance ratios under permutation in the completely randomized design. *J Am Statist Assoc*; 1966; 61: 813–820.
p-dist.

21. Baker FB; LJ Hubert. Inference procedures for ordering theory. *J Educ Statist*; 1977; 2: 217–233.
p-dist.

22. Barbella P; L Denby and JM Glandwehr. Beyond exploratory data analysis: The randomization test. *Math Teacher*; 1990; 83: 144–49.
concept.

23. Barber WC; MV Dayhoff. *Atlas of Protein Sequence and Structure*. Washington DC: National Biomedical Research Foundation; 1972.
application.

24. Barnard GA. Conditionality versus similarity in the analysis of 2 × 2 tables. in *Essays in Honor of CR Rao*. Amsterdam: N Holland; 1982: 59–65.
xtab/concept.

25. Barnard GA. Discussion of paper by MS Bartlett. *J Roy Statist Soc B*; 1963; 25: 294.
estimating p.

26. Barton DE; FN David. The random intersection of two graphs. *Research papers in statistics*. FN David. New York: Wiley; 1966.
p-dist.

27. Barton DE; FN David. Randomization basis for multivariate tests. *Bull Int Statist Inst*; 1961; 39: 455–467.
multivariate.

28. Barton DE; FN David, E Fix, M Merrington and P Mustacchi. Tests for space-time interaction and a power transformation. From Lucien LeCam. Proceedings

5th Berkeley Symposium on Mathematical Statistics and Probability. Berkeley: University of California Press; 1967; IV.
clusters.

29. Basu D. Discussion of Joseph Berkson's paper "In dispraise of the exact test". *J Statist Plan Infer*; 1979; 3: 189–192.
xtab/concept.

30. Basu D. On the relevance of randomization in data analysis (with discussion). in *Survey Sampling and Measurement*. NK Namboodiri, Ed. New York: Academic Press; 1978: 267–339.
concept/limits.

31. Basu D. Randomization analysis of experimental data: The Fisher randomization test. *J Am Statist Assoc*; 1980; 75: 575–582.

32. Bedrick KE; Hill JR. Outlier tests for logistic regression: a conditional approach. *Biometrika*; 1990; 77: 815–827.
logistic regression.

33. Bell CB; KA Doksum. Distribution-free tests of independence. *Annals Math Statist*; 1967; 38: 429–446.
independence/concept/theory.

34. Bell CB; KA Doksum. Some new distribution free statistics. *Annals Math Statist*; 1965; 36: 203–214.

35. Bell CB; JF Donoghue. Distribution-free tests of randomness. *Sankhya* A; 1969; 31: 157–176.
time-series/stationarity/theory.

36. Bell CP; PK Sen. Randomization Procedures. *Nonparametric Methods*. PR Krishnaiah and PK Sen, Editors. Amsterdam: North-Holland; 1984; 4: 1–30.
concept/review.

37. Berkson J. Do the marginals of the 2×2 table contain relevant information respecting the table proportions? *J Statist Prob Inference*; 1979; 3: 193–7.
concept/xtab.

38. Berkson J. In dispraise of the exact test. *J Stat Plan Inf*; 1978; 2: 27–42.
xtab/concept.

39. Berry KJ; KL Kvamme, and PWjr Mielke. Improvements in the permutation test for the spatial analysis of the distribution of artifacts into classes. *Am Antiquity*; 1983; 48: 547–553.
application.

40. Berry KJ; KL Kvamme, and PWjr Mielke. Permutation techniques for the spatial analysis of the distribution of artifacts into classes. *Am Antiquity*; 1980; 45: 55–59.
application.

41. Berry KJ; PWjr Mielke, and RKW Wary. Approximate MRPP *p*-values obtained from four exact moments. *Commun Statist B*; 1986; 15: 581–589.
MRPP/algorithm.

42. Berry KJ; PWjr Mielke. Computation of finite population parameters and approximate probability values of multi-response permutation procedures (MRPP). *Commun Statist B*; 1983; 12: 83–107.
multivariate.

43. Berry KJ; PWjr Mielke. Computation of exact probability values for multi-response permutation procedures (MRPP). *Commun Stat B*; 1984; 13: 417–432.
algorithm/multivariate.

44. Berry KJ; PWjr Mielke. Computation of exact and approximate probability values for a matched-pairs permutation test. *Commun Statist B*; 1985; 14: 229–248.
algorithm/matched-pairs/sign test.

45. Berry KJ; PWjr Mielke, and SG Helmericks. Exact confidence limits for proportions. *Educat Psych Measure*; 1988; 48: 713–716.
    confidence limits/proportions.
46. Besag J; P. Clifford. Generalized Monte Carlo significance tests. *Biometrika*; 1989; 76: 633–42.
    estimating *p*.
47. Besag J; PJ Diggle. Simple Monte Carlo tests for spatial pattern. *App Stat*; 1977; 25: 327–333.
    application.
48. Besag JE. Some methods of statistical analysis for spatial data. *Bull Int Statist Inst*; 1978; 47: 77–92.
    application.
49. Bickel PM; WR Van Zwet. Asymptotic expansion for the power of distribution free tests in the two-sample problem. *Annal Statist*; 1978; 6: 987–1004 (corr 1170–1171).
    power.
50. Bickel PJ. A distribution free version of the Smirnov two-sample test in the multivariate case. *Annals Math Statist*; 1969; 40: 1–23.
    multivariate/conditional *p*-dist.
51. Birch MV. The detection of partial association. *J Roy Statist Soc B*; 1964/5; 26/27: I 313–324 II 1–124.
    xtab.
52. Birnbaum ZW. Computers and unconventional test statistics. in *Reliability and Biometry*. F Presham and RJ Serfing Eds.
    Philadelphia: SIAM; 1974.
53. Boess FG; Balasuvramanian, MJ Brammer and IC Campbell. Stimulation of muscarinic acetylcholine receptors increases synaptosomal free calcium concentration by protein kinase-dependent opening of *L*-type calcium channels. *J Neurochem*; 1990; 55: 230–236.
    application.
54. Boik RJ. The Fisher-Pitman permutation test: a non-robust alternative to the normal theory *F*-test when variances are heterogeneous. *British J Math Stat Psych*; 1987; 40: 26–42.
    misuse.
55. Boos DD; C Browne. Testing for a treatment effect in the presence of nonresponders. *Biometrics*; 1986; 42: 191–197.
    misuse/Wilcoxon/power/nonresponders.
56. Booth JG; RW Butler. Randomization distributions and saddlepoint approximations in general linear models. *Biometrika*; 1990; 77: 787–796.
    saddlepoint/bootstrap.
57. Box GEP; SL Anderson. Permutation theory in the development of robust criteria and the study of departures from assumptions. *J Roy Statist Soc B*; 1955; 17: 1–34 (with discussion).
    p-dist/tests.
58. Boyd MN; PK Sen. Union intersection tests for ordered alternatives in ANOCOVA. *J Amer Statist Assoc*; 1986; 81: 526–32.
    covariate/design.
59. Boyett JM; JJ Shuster. Nonparametric one-sided tests in multivariate analysis with medical applications. *J Amer Statist Assoc*; 1977; 72: 665–668.
    application/multivariate.
60. Bradbury IS. Analysis of variance vs randomization tests: a comparison (with discussion by White and Still). *Brit J Math Stat Psych*; 1987; 40: 177–195.
    p-group/robust/design.

61. Bradbury IS. Approximations to permutation distributions in the completely randomized design. *Commun Statist T-M A*; 1988; 17: 543–55.
asymptotic.

62. Bradley JV. *Distribution Free Statistical Tests*. New Jersey: Prentice-Hall; 1968.
concept/tests.

63. Bradley RA; S Elton. Perspectives from a weather modification experiment. *Commun Statist A*; 1980; 9: 1941–61.
application.

64. Breslow NE; NE Day. *I. Analysis of Case Control Studies. II. Design and Analysis of Cohort Studies*. New York: Oxford University Press; 1980, 1987.
test/p-dist/estimation/logistic models.

65. Brockwell PJ; PWjr Mielke. Asymptotic distributions of matched-pair permutation statistics based on distance measures. *Austral J Statist*; 1984; 26: 30–38.
asymptotic/rank tests/matched-pairs.

66. Brockwell PJ; PWjr Mielke, and J Robinson. On non-normal invariance principles for multi-response permutation procedures. *Austral J Statist*; 1982; 24: 33–41.
theory.

67. Bross IDJ. Taking a covariable into account. *J Am Statist Assoc*; 1964; 59: 725–736.
application/covariate.

68. Brown BM. Cramer-von Mises distributions and permutation tests. *Biometrika*; 1982; 69: 619–624.
theory.

69. Brown BM; TP Hettmansperger. Affine invariant rank methods in the bivariate location model. *J Roy Statist Soc B*; 1987; 49: 301–310.
rank/bivariate/location/application.

70. Brown CC; TR Fears. Exact significance levels for multiple binomial testing with applications to carcinogenicity screens. *Biometrics*; 1981; 37: 763–774.
exact/simultaneous inference.

71. Bryant EH. Morphometric adaptation of the housefly, Musa domestica L., in the United States. *Evolution*; 1977; 31: 580–596.
application/cluster.

72.. Buckland ST; PH Garthwaite. Quantifying precision of mark-recapture estimates using the bootstrap and related methods. *Biometrics*; 1991; 47: 225–268.
estimation.

73. Buonaccorsi JP. A note on confidence intervals for proportions in finite populations. *Amer Stat*; 1987; 41: 215–218.
proportions.

74. Busby DG. Effects of aerial spraying of fenithrothion on breeding white-throated sparrows. *J Appl Ecology*; 1990; 27: 745–755.
application.

75. Cade BS; RW Hoffman. Winter use of Douglas-fir forests by blue grouse in Colorado. *J Wildlife Man*; 1990; 27: 743–755.
application.

76. Casagrande JJ; MC Pike, PG Smith. The power function of the exact test for comparing two binomial distributions. *App Statist*; 1978; 27: 176–181.
power/exact test/cross-tabulation.

77. Chapelle JP; A Albert, JP Smeets, C Heusghem, and HE Kulberts. Effect of the hyptoglobin phenotype on the size of a mycocardial infarct. *New Eng J Med*; 1982; 307: 457–463.
application.

78. Chatterjee SK; PK Sen. *Calcutta Statist Assoc Bull*; 1973; 22: 13–50.
    robust.
79. Chatterjee SK; PK Sen. Nonparametric tests for the bivariate two-sample location problem. *Calcutta Statist Assoc Bull*; 1964; 13: 18–58.
    location/bivariate.
80. Chatterjee SK; PK Sen. Nonparametric tests for the multivariate, multisample location problem. *Essays in Probability and Statistics in memory of SN Roy*. RC Bose etal. Eds. Chapel Hill NC: University of North Carolina Press; 1966.
    tests/multivar.
81. Chen XR. Large sample theory of permutation tests in the case of a randomized block design. *J Wuhan University*, Natural Science Edition; 1983; 4: 1–12.
    clt.
82. Chen XR. Two problems of linear permutation statistics. *Acta Math Appl Sinica*; 1981; 4: 342–355.
    concept.
83. Chen XR. A two-sample permutation test with heterogeneous blocks. *Wuhan Daxue Xuebao*; 1980; 4: 1–14.
    test/exact.
84. Chernoff H, IR Savage. Asymptotic normality and efficiency of certain non-parametric test statistics. *Annal Math Statist*; 29.
    asymptotic.
85. Chung JH; DAS Fraser. Randomization tests for a multivariate two-sample problem. *J Am Statist Assoc*; 1958; 53: 729–735.
    multivariate/algorithm/application/choose.
86. Clark RM. A randomization test for the comparison of ordered sequences. *Mathem Geol*; 1989; 21: 429–442.
    application/chose.
87. Cliff AD; JK Ord. Evaluating the percentage points of a spatial autocorrelation coefficient. *Geog Analysis*; 1971; 3: 51–62.
    cluster.
88. Cliff AD; JK Ord. *Spatial Autocorrelation*. London: Pion; 1973.
    application.
89. Cliff AD; JK Ord. *Spatial Processes: Models and Applications*. London: Pion Ltd; 1981.
    space-time/application.
90. Cohen A. Unbiasedness of tests for homogenity. *Annal Statist*; 1987; 15: 805–816.
    theory.
91. Collier RO jr; FB Baker. The randomization distribution of *F*-ratios for the split-plot design—an empirical investigation. *Biometrika*; 1963; 50: 431–438.
    p-dist/design/simulation.
92. Collier RO, jr; FB Baker. Some Monte Carlo results on the power of the *F*-test under permutation in the simple randomized block design. *Biometrika*; 1966; 53: 199–203.
    simulation/power/design.
93. Collins MF. A permutation test for planar regression. *Austral J Statist*; 1987; 29: 303–308.
    test.
94. Conlon M; RG Thomas. AS280, Power function for Fisher's exact test. *Applied Statistics*; 1993; 42: 258–260.
95. Conover WJ. *Practical Nonparametric Statistics*. New York: Jonn Wiley & Sons; 1971.
    test.
96. Constanzo CM; LJ Hubert and RG Golledge. A higher moment for spatial statistics. Geographical Analysis; 1983; 15: 347–351.
    application/moments.

97. Cornfeld J. A statistical problem arising from retrospective studies. *Proceedings of 3rd Berkeley Symposium on Mathematical Statistics and Probability*. J. Neyman. Ed. Berkeley: University of California Press; 1956; 4: 135–138.

98. Cornfield J. On samples from finite populations. *J Am Statist Assoc*; 1944; 39: 236–239.
concept.

99. Cornfield J; JW Tukey. Average values of mean squares in factorials. *Annal Math Statist*; 1956; 27: 907–949.
p-dist/concept/design.

100. Cory-Slechta DA. Exposure duration modalities, the effects of low-level lead on fixed interval performances. *Neurotoxicology*; 1990; 11: 427–442.
application.

101. Cory–Slechta DA; B Weiss and C Cox. Tissue distribution of Pb in adult vs old rats: a pilot study. *Toxicology*; 1989; 59: 139–150.
application.

102. Cotton JW. Even better than before. *Contemp Psychol*; 1973; 18: 168–169.

103. Cox DF; O Kempthorne. Randomization tests for comparing survival curves. *Biometrics*; 1963; 19: 307–317.
tests/application.

104. Cox DR. Interpretation of nonadditivity in Latin Square. *Biometrika*; 1958; 45: 69–73.
design.

105. Cox DR. A note on weighted randomization. *Annal Math Statist*; 1956; 27: 1144–1150.
p-dist/design.

106. Cox DR. A remark on randomization in clinical trials. *Utilitas Math*; 1982; 21A: 242–252.
concept/application/clinical trials/restriction.

107. Cox DR; PAW Lewis. *The Statistical Analysis of Series of Events*. New York: Wiley & Sons; 1966.
independence.

108. Cox DR; EJ Shell. *Analysis of Binary Data* 2 Ed. London: Chapman-Hall; 1989.
xtab.

109. Cox MAA; RL Plackett. Small samples in contingency tables. *Biometrika*; 1980; 67: 1–13.
algorithm/xtab.

110. Crump KS; RB Howe, and RL Kodell. Permutation tests for detecting teratogenic effects. Krewski D; C Franklin, editors. *Statistics in Toxicology*. New York: Gordon and Breach Science Publishers; 1990: 347–375.
choice/teratogenic/application.

111. D'Abadie C; F Proschan. Stochastic versions of rearrangement inequalities. YL Tong, Editor. *Inequalities in Statistics and Probability*. Hayward CA: IMS; 1984: 4–12.
algorithm.

112. D'Agostino RB; W Chase and A Belanger. The appropriateness of some common procedures for testing the equality of two independent binomial populations. *Am Statistician*; 1988; 42: 198–202.
xtab.

113. Daniels HE. Relation between measures of correlation in the universe of sample permutations. *Biometrika*; 1944; 33: 129–135.
p-dist/dependence.

114. Dansie BR. A note on permutation probabilities. *J Roy Statist Soc B*; 1983; 45: 22–24.
p-dist.

115. David FN. Measurement of diversity. *Proceedings 6th Berkeley Symposium*; 1971; 1: 631–648.

116. David FN; Barton DE. *Combinatorial Chance*. New York: Hafner; 1962.
    concept.

117. David FN; DE Barton. Two space-time interaction tests for epidemicity. *Brit J Prevent and Soc Med*; 1966; 20: 44–48.
    clustering.

118. Davis AW. On certain ratio statistics in weather modification experiments. *Technometrics*; 1979; 21: 283–290.
    p-dist/power/application.

119. Davis AW; TP Speed. An Edgeworth expansion for the distribution of the *F*-ratio under the randomization model for the randomized block design. SS Gupta and JO Berger. *Statistical Decision Theory and Related Topics*. New York: Springer Verlag; 1988; 2: 119–129.
    asymptotic.

120. Davis LJ. Exact tests for 2 × 2 contingency tables. *Am Statistician*; 1986; 40: 139–140.
    xtab.

121. Denker M; ML Puir. Asymptotic behavior of multi-response permutation procedures. *Adv Appl Math*; 1988; 9: 200–210.
    asymptotic/MMRP.

122. Dennis AS; JR Miller, DE Cain, RL Schwaller. Evaluation by Monte Carlo tests of effects of cloud seeding on growing season rainfall in North Dakota. *J App Meteorol*, 1975; 14: 959–964.
    application.

123. Deutsch SJ; BW Schmeiser. The power of paired sample *t*-tests. *Naval Res Logistics Quar*; 1982; 29: 635–649.
    power/theory.

124. Deutsch ST; BW Schmeiser. The computation of the component randomization test for paired comparisons. *J Quality Technol*; 1983; 15: 94–98.
    matched pairs.

125. Diaconis P; B Efron. Computer intensive methods in statistics. *Scientific American*; 1983; 48: 116–130.
    tests.

126. Diaconis P; RL Graham. Spearman's footrule as a measure of disarray. *J Roy Statist Soc B*; 1972; 39: 262–268.
    metric.

127. Dietz EJ. Permutation tests for the association between two distance matricies. *Systemic Zool*; 1983; 32: 21–26.
    Mantel/application.

128. Diggle PJ. *Statistical Analysis of Spatial Point Patterns*. London: Academic Press; 1983.
    application.

129. Donegani, M. An adaptive and powerful test. *Biometrika*; 1991; 78: 930–933.
    adaptive/matched-pairs.

130. Donegani M. Asymptotic and approximate distribution of a statistic obtained by resampling with and without replacement. *Statist and Probab Lett*; 1991; 11: 181–183.
    bootstrap.

131. Donner A. Odds ratio inference with dependent data: a relationship between two procedures. *Biometrika*; 74.
    xtab.

132. Doolittle RF. Similar amino acid sequences: chance or common ancestory. *Science*; 1981; 214: 149–159.
     application.
133. Douglas ME; JA Endler. Quantitative matrix comparisons in ecological and evolutionary investigations. *J Theoret Biol*; 1982; 99: 777–795.
     Mantel/application.
134. Draper NR; DM Stoneman. Testing for the inclusion of variables in linear regression by a randomization technique. *Technometrics*; 1966; 8: 695–699.
     trend.
135. Dwass M. Modified randomization tests for non-parametric hypotheses. *Annal Math Statist*; 1957; 28: 181–187.
     algorithm/power/Monte Carlo.
136. Dwass M. On the asymptotic normality of some statistics used in nonparametric tests. *Annal Math Statist*; 1955; 26: 334–339.
     clt.
137. Easterling RG. Randomization and statistical inference. *Commun Statist*; 1975; 4: 723–735.
     power.
138. Edelman D. Bounds for a nonparametric t-table. *Biometrika*; 1986, 73: 242–243.
     asymptotic.
139. Eden T; F Yates. On the validity of Fisher's z test when applied to an actual sample of nonnormal data. *J Agric Sci*; 1933; 23: 6–16.
     robust.
140. Edgington ES. Approximate randomization tests. *J Psych*; 1969; 72: 143–149.
     concept/restricted.
141. Edgington ES. Hypothesis testing without fixed levels of significance. *J Psych*; 1970; 76: 109–115.
     concept.
142. Edgington ES. Overcoming obstacles to single-subject experimentation. *J Educ Statist*; 1980; 5: 261–267.
     single-subject.
143. Edgington ES. Randomization tests. *J Psych*; 1964; 57: 445–449.
     review.
144. Edgington ES. Randomization tests for one-subject operant experiments. *J Psych*; 1975; 90: 57–68.
     concept.
145. Edgington ES. Randomization tests for predicted trends. *Canad Psych Rev*; 1975; 16: 49–53.
     trend test.
146. Edgington ES. *Randomization Tests*. New York: Marcel Dekker; 1980, 1987.
     tests/review.
147. Edgington ES. The role of permutation groups in randomization tests. *J Educ Stat*; 1983; 8: 121–145.
     concept.
148. Edgington ES. Statistical inference and nonrandom samples. *Psychol Bull*; 1966; 66: 485–487.
     concept.
149. Edgington ES. Statistics and single-case analysis. Miltersen, RM Eisler, and PM Miller. *Progress in Behavior Modification*. New York: Academic Press; 1984; 16.
     single-case.
150. Edgington ES. Validity of randomization tests for one-subject experiments. *J Educ Stat*; 1980; 5: 235–251.
     test/repeated measures.

151. Edgington ES; G Ezinga. Randomization tests and outlier scores. *J Psych*; 1978; 99: 259–262.
      concept/robust.
152. Edgington ES; AP Gore. Randomization tests for censored survival distributions. *Biometrical J*; 1986; 28: 673–681.
      censored.
153. Edgington ES; AR Strain. A computer program for randomization tests for predicted trends. *Behav Res Meth and Instrum*; 1976; 8: 470–470.
      trends/program.
154. Edgington ES; AR Strain. Randomization tests: computer time requirements. *J Psychol*; 1973; 85: 89–95.
      algorithm.
155. Efron B. Forcing sequential experiments to be balanced. *Biometrika*; 1971; 58: 403–417.
      clinical trials.
156. Efron B. Three examples of computer intensive statistical inference. *Sankhya* A; 1988; 50: 338–362.
      restricted.
157. Elliot RD; KJ Brown. The Santa Barbara II project—downwind effects. *International Conference on Weather Modification*;
      Preprint: 179–184.
      application/comparison of tests.
158. Entsuah AR. Randomization procedures for analyzing clinical trend data with treatment related withdrawls. *Commun Statist A*; 1990; 19: 3859–3880.
      missing/clinical/choose/application.
159. Erdos P; A Renyi. On a central limit theorem for samples from a finite population. *Publ Math Inst Hung Acad Sci*; 1959; 4: 49–61.
      clt.
160. Fan CT; ME Muller and I Rezucha. Development of sampling plans by using sequential (item by item) selection techniques and digital computers. *J Am Statist Assoc*; 1962; 57: 387–402.
      algorithm.
161. Fang KT. The limit distribution of linear permutation statistics and its applications. *Acta Math Appl Sinica*; 1981; 4: 69–82.
      clt.
162. Faris PD; RS Sainsbury. The role of the Pontis Oralis in the generation of RSA activity in the hippocampus of the guinea pig. *Psychol and Behav*; 1990; 47: 1193–1199.
      application.
163. Farrar DA; KS Crump. Exact statistical tests for any carcinogenic effect in animal assays. *Fund Appl Toxicol*;1988; 11: 652–663.
      combinations of tests/application.
164. Farrar DA; KS Crump. Exact statistical tests for any carcinogenic effect in animal assays. II age adjusted tests. *Fund Appl Toxicol*; 1991; 15: 710–721.
      combinations of tests/application.
165. Fears TR; RE Tarone and KC Chu. False-positive and false-negative rates for carcinogenicity screens. *Cancer Research*; 1977; 37: 1941–1945.
      exact/applicatlon.
166. Feinstein AR. *Clinical Biostatistics*. St Louis: Mosby; 1972.
      application.
167. Feinstein AR. Clinical biostatistics XXIII. The role of randomization in sampling, testing, allocation, and credulous idolatry (part 2). *Clinical Pharm*; 1973; 14: 989–1009.
      concept.

168. Finch PD. Description and analogy in the practice of statistics (with disc). *Biometrika*; 1979; 66: 195–205.
     exploratory/concept/rank tests.
169. Finney DJ. Fisher-Yates test of significance in 2×2 contingency table. *Biometrika*; 1948; 35: 145–156.
     cross-tab.
170. Fisher, RA. Coefficient of racial likeness and the future of craniometry. *J Royal Anthrop Soc*; 1936; 66: 57–63.
     p-dist/concept.
171. Fisher, RA. *The Design of Experiments* 6th Ed. New York: Hafner; 1951.
     concept/*p*-dist.
172. Fisher RA. The logic of inductive inference (with discussion). *J Roy Statist Soc A*; 1934; 98: 39–54.
     exact test/concept.
173. Fisher RA. *Statistical Methods for Research Workers*. Edinburgh: Oliver & Boyd; 1936.
     concept.
174. Ford RD; LV Colom and BH Bland. The classification of medial septum-diagonal band cells as theta-on or theta-off in relation to hippo campal EEG states. *Brain Research*; 1989; 493: 269–282.
     application.
175. Forsythe AB; L Engleman, and R Jennrich. A stopping rule for variable selection in multivariate regression. *J Am Statist Assoc*; 1973; 68: 75–77.
     regression/*p*-dist.
176. Forsythe AB; HS Frey. Tests of significance from survival data. *Computers and Biomed Res*; 1970; 3: 124–132. Monte Carlo.
177. Foutz RN; DR Jensen, and GW Anderson. Multiple comparisons in the randomization analysis of designed experiments with growth curve responses. *Biometrics*; 1985; 41: 29–37.
     application/growth curve/multiple comparisons.
178. Foutz RV. A method for constructing exact tests from test statistics that have unknown null distributions. *J Statist* Comput Simul; 1980; 10: 187–193.
     concept.
179. Foutz RV. Simultaneous randomization tests. *Biometrical J*; 1984; 26: 655–663.
     multiple comparisons.
180. Frank, D; RJ Trzos, and P Good. Evaluating drug-induced chromosome alterations. *Mutation Res*; 1978; 56: 311–317.
     application.
181. Fraser DW. Clustering of disease in population units: an exact test and its asymptotic version. *Amer J Epidemiol*; 1983; 118: 732–739.
     choice/application.
182. Fraumeni JF; FP Li. Hodgkin's disease in childhood: an epidemiological study. *J Nat Cancer Inst*; 1969; 42: 681–691.
     Mantel/application.
183. Freedman D; D Lane. The empirical distribution of Fourier coefficients. *Annal Statist*; 1980; 8: 1244–1251.
     p-dist.
184. Freedman D; D Lane. Nonstochastic interpretation of reported significance levels. *J Bus Econ Stat*; 1983; 1: 292–298.
     covariate/design.
185. Freedman L. Using permutation tests and bootstrap confidence limits to analyze repeated events data. *Controlled Clinical Trials*; 1989; 10: 129–141.
     application/repeated measures.

186. Freeman GH; JH Halton. Note on an exact treatment of contingency, goodness of fit, and other problems of significance. *Biometrika*; 1951; 38: 141–149. xtab/misuse.

187. Friedman JH; LC Rafsky. Multivariate generalizations of the Wald-Wolfowitz and Smirnov two-sample test. *Annal Statist*; 1979; 7: 697–717. trend/multivariate.

188. Gabriel KR. Some statistical issues in weather experimentation. *Commun Statist A*; 1979; 8: 975–1015. application/restricted/historical regression/multiple comparisons.

189. Gabriel KR; P Feder. On the distribution of statistics suitable for evaluating rainfall simulation experiments. *Technometrics*; 1969; 11: 149–160. application.

190. Gabriel KR; WJ Hall. Rerandomization inference on regression and shift effects: Computationally feasible methods. *J Am Statist Assoc*; 1983; 78: 827–836. confidence-intervals/algorithm.

191. Gabriel KR; CF Hsu. Evaluation of the power of rerandomization tests, with application to weather modification experiments. *J Am Statist Assoc*; 1983; 78: 766–775. power/application.

192. Gabriel KR; RR Sokal. A new statistical approach to geographical variation analysis. *Systematic Zoology*; 1969; 18: 259–70. Mantel.

193. Gail MH; WY Tan, and S. Piantadosi. Tests for no treatment effect in randomized clinical trials. *Biometrika*; 1988; 75: 57–64. covariate/design.

194. Gans LP; CA Robertson. Distributions of Goodman and Kruskal's Gamma and Spearman's Rho in 2×2 tables for small and moderate sample sizes. *J Am Statist Assoc*; 1981; 76: 942–946. exact test/cross-tab/Monte Carlo.

195. Geary RC. Metron; 1927; 7: 83. concept.

196. Gerig TM. A multivariate extension of Friedman's chi-square test. *J Am Statist Assoc*; 1969; 64: 1595–1608. multivariate/ranks/design.

197. Gerig TM. A multivariate extension of Friedman's chi-square test with random covariates. *J Am Statist Assoc*; 1975; 70: 443–447. application/asymptotic/design/multivariate/covariate.

198. Ghosh MN. Asymptotic distributions of serial statistics and applications to nonparametric tests of hypotheses. *Annal Math Statist*; 1954; 25: 218–251. asymptotic/independence/power.

199. Gill DS; M Siotani. On randomization in the multivariate analysis of variance. *J Statist Plan Infer*; 1987; 17: 217–226. design/MANOVA/Wilk's statistic/p-dist.

200. Glass AG; N Mantel. Lack of time-space clustering of childhood leukemia, Los Angeles County 1960–64. *Cancer Research*; 1969; 29: 1995–2001. Mantel/application.

201. Glass AG; N Mantel, FW Gunz, and GFS Spears. Time-space clustering of childhood leukemia in New Zealand. *J Nat Cancer Inst*; 1971; 47: 329–336. application.

202. Glick BJ. Tests for space-time clustering used in cancer research. *Geographical Analy*; 1979; 11: 202–208. concept.

203. Goldberg P; F Leffert, M Gonzales, L Gorgenola, and GO Zerbe. Intraveneous

aminophylline in asthma: A comparison of two methods of administration in children. *Am J of Diseases and Children*; 1980; 134: 12–18.
application.

204. Good IJ. On the analysis of symmetric Dirichlet distributions and their mixtures to contingency tables. *Annal of Statist*; 1976; 4: 1159–89.
tails/xtab.

205. Good P. Almost most powerful tests for composite alternatives. *Communications in statistics—theory and methods*; 1989; 18: 1913–1925.
application/test.

206. Good P. Most powerful tests for use in matched pair experiments when data may be censored. *J Statist Comp Simul*; 1991; 38: 57–63.
matched-pairs/power/algorithm/censored/bootstrap.

207. Good P. Review of Edgington's Randomization Tests. *J Statist Comput Simul*; 1980; 11: 157–160.
power.

208. Good P; P Kemp. Almost most powerful test for censored data. *Randomization*; 1969; 2: 25–33.
application/censored.

209. Good, PI. Detection of a treatment effect when not all experimental subjects respond to treatment. *Biometrics*; 1979; 35: 483–489.
application/robust.

210. Good PI. Globally almost powerful tests for censored data. *Nonparametric Statistics*; 1992; 1: 253–262.
censored data/test/concepts.

211. Goodall DW. Contingency tables and computers. *Praximetric*; 1968; 9: 113–119.
xtab/program.

212. Graubard BI; EL Korn. Choice of column scores for testing independence in ordered 2 by K contingency tables. *Biometrics*; 1987; 43: 471–476.
choice/ordered classifications/xtabs.

213. Graves GW; Whinston AB Whinston. An algorithm for the quadratic assignment probability. *Management Science*; 1970; 17: 453–471.
algorithm/Mantel.

214. Green BF. Review of Edgington's Randomization Tests. *J Am Statist Assoc*; 1981; 76: 495.
review.

215. Haber M. A comparison of some conditional and unconditional exact tests for 2×2 contingency tables. *Commun Statist A*; 1987; 18: 147–156.
power/xtab.

216. Hack HRB. An empirical investigation into the distribution of the F-ratio in samples from two non-normal populations. *Biometrika*; 1958; 45: 260–265.
robust/simulation/p-dist.

217. Hajek J. Asymptotic normality of simple linear rank statistics under alternatives. *Annal Math Statist*; 1968; 39: 325–346.
clt/power.

218. Hajek J. Limiting distributions in simple random sampling from a finite population. *Publ Math Inst Hung Acad Sci*; 1960; 5: 361–374.
clt.

219. Hajek J. Some extensions of the Wald-Wolfowitz-Noether theorem. *Annal Math Statist*; 1961; 32: 506–523.
clt.

220. Hajek J; Z Sidak. *Theory of Rank Tests*. New York: Academic Press; 1967.
p-dist/ranks.

221. Halter JH. A rigorous derivation of the exact contingency formula. *Proc Cambridge Phil Soc*; 1969; 65: 527–530.
xtab/exact test/*p*-dist.

222. Hampel FR, EM Ronchetti, PJ Rousseeuw, WA Stahel. *Robust Statistics; The Approach Based on Influence Functions.* New York: John Wiley; 1966.
robust/flaws and misuse.

223. Henery RJ. Permutation probabilities for gamma random variables. *J Appl Probab*; 1983; 20: 822–834.
gamma.

224. Henze N. A multivariate two-sample test based on the number of nearest neighbor coincidence. *Annal Statist*; 1988; 16: 772–783.
multivariate.

225. Hiatt WR; DC Fradl, GO Zerbe, RL Byyny, and AS Niels. Comparative effects of selective and nonselective beta blockers on the peripheral circulation. *Clinic Pharmacology and Therapeutics*; 1983; 35: 12–18.
application.

226. Highton R. Comparison of microgeographic variation in morphological and electrophoretic traits. Hecht MK, Steer WC, & B Wallace, editors. *Evolutionary Biology.* New York: Plenum; 1977; 10: 397–436.
Mantel/application.

227. Hirji KF; CR Mehta, and NR Patel. Computing distributions for exact logistic regression. *J Am Statist Assoc*; 1987; 82: 1110–1117.
algorithm/*p*-dist.

228. Hirji KF; CR Mehta, and NR Patel. Exact inference for matched case-control studies. *Biometrics*; 1988; 44: 803–814.
case-control.

229. Ho ST; LHY Chen. An Lp bound for the remainder in a combinatorial central limit theorem. *Annal Probability*; 1978; 6: 231–249.
asymptotic/theory.

230. Hoeffding, W. Combinatorial central limit theorem. *Annal Math Statist*; 1951; 22: 556–558.
clt.

231. Hoeffding W. The large-sample power of tests based on permutations of observations. *Annal Math Statist*; 1952; 23: 169–192.
power.

232. Hollander M; E Pena. Nonparametric tests under restricted treatment assigment rules. *J Am Statist Assoc*; 1988; 83: 1144–1151.
tests/restricted/algorithm.

233. Hollander M; J Sethuraman. Testing for agreement between two groups of judges. *Biometrika*; 1978; 65: 403–412.
application/correlation.

234. Hollander M; DA Wolfe. *Nonparametric Methods in Statistics.* New York: Wiley; 1973.
concept/tests.

235. Hope ACA. A modified Monte Carlo significance test procedure. *J Roy Statist Soc B*; 1968; 30: 582–598.
test.

236. Howard, M (pseud); P Good. Randomization in the analysis of experiments and clinical trials. *American Laboratory*; 1981; 13: 98–102.
review.

237. Huber PJ. A robust version of the probability ratio test. *Annal Math Statist*; 1965; 36: 1753–1758.
robust.

238. Hubert LJ. *Assignment Methods in Combinatorial Data Analysis*. NY: Marcel Dekker; 1987.
cluster.

239. Hubert LJ. Combinatorial data analysis: Association and partial association. *Psychometrika*; 1985; 50: 449–467.
correlation/partial correlation/spatial dist.

240. Hubert LJ. Evaluating object set partitions. *J Verbal Learn Behavior*; 1976; 15: 459–470.
p-dist/classification.

241. Hubert LJ. Generalized proximity function comparisons. *Brit J Math Stat Psych*; 1978a; 31: 179–192.
Mantel/application.

242. Hubert LJ. Generalized concordance. *Psychometrika*; 1979; 44: 3–20.
matrix concordance/multivariate 0–1.

243. Hubert LJ. Matching methods in the analysis of cross-classification. *Psychometrika*; 1979; 44: 21–41.
scale agreement.

244. Hubert LJ. Nonparametric tests for patterns in geographic variation: possible generalizations. *Geog Anal*; 1978b; 10: 86–88.
Mantel.

245. Hubert LJ. Seriation using asymmetric proximity measures. *Brit J Math Stat Psych*; 1976; 29: 32–52.
dependence/application.

246. Hubert LJ; FB Baker. Analyzing distinctive features confusion matrix. *J Educ Statist*; 1977; 2: 79–98.
concept.

247. Hubert LJ; FB Baker. The comparison and fitting of given classification schemes. *J Math Psychol*; 1977; 16: 233–253.
Mantel.

248. Hubert LJ; FB Baker. Data analysis by single-link and complete-link hierarchical clustering. *J Educ Statist*; 1976; 1: 87–111.
test/p-dist.

249. Hubert LJ; FB Baker. Evaluating the conformity of sociometric measurements. *Psychometrika*; 1978; 43: 31–42.
application.

250. Hubert LJ; RG Golledge, and CM Costanzo. Analysis of variance procedures based on a proximity measure between subjects. *Psych Bull*; 1982; 91: 424–430.
Mantel/design.

251. Hubert LJ; RG Golledge, and CM Costanzo. Generalized procedures for evaluating spatial autocorrelation. *Geog Anal*; 1981; 13: 224–233.
application.

252. Hubert LJ; RG Golledge, CM Costanzo, and N Gale. Measuring association between spatially defined variables: An alternative procedure. *Geog Anal*; 1985; 17: 36–46.
spatial autocorrelation.

253. Hubert LJ; RG Golledge, CM Costanzo, N Gale, and WC Halperin. Nonparametric tests for directional data. Bahrenberg G, Fischer M & P Nijkamp, editors. *Recent developments in spatial analysis: Methodology, measurement, models*. Aldershot UK: Gower; 1984: 171–190.
Mantel/spatial analysis.

254. Hubert LJ; JR Levin. General statistical framework for assessing categorical clustering in free recall. *Psych Bull*; 1976; 83: 1072–1080.
application/p-dist/classification.

255. Hubert LJ; JR Levin. Inference models for categorical clustering. *Psych Bull*; 1976; 83: 878–887.
     xtab.
256. Hubert LJ; J Schultz. Maximum likelihood paired comparison ranking and quadratic assessment. *Biometrika*; 1975; 62: 655–660.
     algorithm.
257. Hubert LJ; J Schultz. Quadratic assignment as a general data analysis strategy. *Brit J Math Stat Psych*; 1976; 29: 190–241.
     Mantel.
258. Ingenbleek JF. Tests simultanes de permutation des rangs pour bruit-blanc multivarie. *Statist Anal Donnees*; 1981; 6: 60–65.
     simultaneous/tests/multivariate.
259. Irony TZ; CAB Pereira. Exact tests for equality of two proportions: Fisher vs Bayes. *J Statist Comput Simul*; 1986; 25: 83–114.
     concept/xtab/significance level/power.
260. Iyer HK; K Berry, and PWJr Mielke. Computation of finite population parameters and approximate probability values for multi-response randomized block permutation procedures (MRPP). *Commun Statist B*; 1983; 12: 479–499.
     MRPP/multivariate/moments.
261. Jackson DA. Ratios in acquatic sciences: Statistical shortcomings with mean depth and the morphoedaphic index. *Canad J Fisheries and Acquatic Sci*; 1990; 47: 1788–1795.
     application/concept.
262. Janssen A. Conditional rank tests for randomly censored data. *Annals of Statistics*; 1991; 19: 1434–1456.
     censor.
263. Jennrich RI. A note on the behaviour of the log rank permutation test under unequal censoring. *Biometrika*: 1983; 70: 133–137.
     flaws.
264. Jennrich RI. Some exact tests for comparing survival curves in the presence of unequal right censoring. *Biometrika*; 1984; 71: 57–64.
     conditional.
265. Jin MZ. On the multisample pemutation test when the experimental units are nonuniform and random experimental errors exist. *J System Sci Math Sci*; 1984; 4: 117–127, 236–243.
     tests.
266. Jockel KH. Finite sample properties and asymptotic efficiency of Monte Carlo tests. *Annal Statistics*; 1986; 14: 336–347.
     power/Monte Carlo.
267. Jogdeo K. Asymptotic normality in nonparametric methods. *Annal Math Statist*; 1968; 39: 905–922.
     asymptotic/rank/U-statistics/theory.
268. John RD; Robinson J. Edgeworth expansions for the power of permutation tests. *Annal of Statistics*; 1983; 11: 625–631.
     power.
269. John RD; J Robinson. Significance levels and confidence intervals for randomization tests. *J Statist Comput and Simul*; 1983; 16: 161–173.
     confidence intervals.
270. Johnson NL. Theoretical considerations regarding HRB Hack's system of randomization for crossclassifications. *Biometrika*; 1958; 45: 265–266.
     xtab.
271. Jones JS; RK Selander, and GD Schnell. *Biol J Linnean Society*; 1980; 14: 359.
     Mantel/application.
272. Kalbfleisch JD. Likelihood methods and nonparametric tests. *J Am Statist*

Assoc; 1978; 73: 167–170.
marginal likelihood/*p*-dist.

273. Kalbfleisch JD; RL Prentice. *Statistical Analysis of Failure Time Data.* New York: John Wiley & Sons; 1980.
p-dist/bootstraping.

274. Karlin S; G Ghandour, F Ost, S Tauare, and K Korph. New approaches for computer analysis of DNA sequences. *Proc Nat Acad Sci*, USA; 1983; 80: 5660–5664.
application.

275. Karlin S; PT Williams. Permutation methods for the structured exploratory data analysis (SEDA) of familial trait values. *Amer J Human Genetics*; 1984; 36.
application/choice.

276. Kazdin AE. Obstacles in using randomization tests in single-case experiments. *J Educ Statist*; 1980; 5: 253–260.
repeated measures/misuse.

277. Kazdin AE. Statistical analysis for single-case experimental designs. in *Single-Case Experimental Design: Strategies for Studying Behavioral Change.* M Hersen and DH Barlow, Eds. New York: Pergamon; 1976.
concept/repeated measures.

278. Keller-McNulty S; JJ Higgens. Effect of tail weight and outliers on power and type I error of robust permutation tests for location. *Commun Stat—Theory and Methods*; 1987; 16: 17–35.
robust/power.

279. Kelly ME. Application of the theory of combinatorial chance to the estimation of significance of clustering in free recall. *Brit J Math Stat Psych*; 1973; 26: 270–280.
applic.

280. Kempthorne O. Comments on paper by PD Frich. *Biometrika*; 1979; 66: 206–207.
concept.

281. Kempthorne O. *Design and Analysis of Experiments.* New York: Wiley; 1952.
p-dist/tests.

282. Kempthorne O. In dispraise of the exact test: reactions. *J Statist Plan Infer*; 1979; 3: 199–213.
xtab/concept.

283. Kempthorne O. Inference from experiments and randomization. *A Survey of Statistical Design and Linear Models.* JN Srivastava, Editor. Amsterdam: North Holland; 1975: 303–332.
concept.

284. Kempthorne O. The randomization theory of experimental inference. *J Am Statist Assoc*; 1955; 50: 946–967.
concept/*p*-dist.

285. Kempthorne O. Some aspects of experimental inference. *J Am Statist Assoc*; 1966; 61: 11–34.
concept.

286. Kempthorne O. Why randomize? *J Statist Prob Infer*; 1977; 1: 1–26.
concept.

287. Kempthorne O; TE Doerfler. The behavior of some significance tests under experimental randomization. *Biometrika*; 1969; 56: 231–248.
power/rank/confidence intervals.

288. Kempthorne O; G Zyskind, S Addelman, T Throckmorton, and R White. Analysis of variance procedures: Report ARL149, Aeronautical Research Laboratory, USAF; 1961.
asymptotic/*p*-dist/design.

289. Kendall MG; A Stuart, and JK Ord. *Advanced Theory of Statistics*. London: Charles Griffin & Co; 1977 (4th Edition).
     design.
290. Khan KA; DS Tracy. Fourth exact moment results for MRPP tests with 2 or 3 treatments. *Commun Statist A*; 1991; 20 3863–3877.
291. Klauber MR. Space-time clustering tests for more than two samples. *Biometrics*; 1975; 31: 719–726.
     application/*p*-dist.
292. Klauber MR. Two-sample randomization tests for space-time clustering. *Biometrics*; 1971; 27: 129–142.
     application/*p*-dist.
293. Klauber MR; Mustacchi. Space-time clustering of childhood leukemia in San Francisco. *Cancer Research*; 1970; 30: 1969–1973.
     Mantel/application.
294. Kleinbaum DB; LL Kupper, and LE Chambless. Logistic regression analysis of epidemiologic data: theory and practice. *Commun Statist A*; 1982; 11: 485–547.
     logistic/application.
295. Kolchin VF; VP Christyakov. On a combinatorial central limit theorem. *Theor Prob & Appl*; 1973; 18: 728–739.
     theory/asymptotic/clt.
296. Koziol JA; DA Maxwell, M Fukushima, A Colmer, and YH Pilch. A distribution-free test for tumor-growth curve analyses with applications to an animal tumor immunotherapy experiment. *Biometrics*; 1981; 37: 383–390.
     multivariate/application/*p*-dist.
297. Krewski D; J Brennan, and M Bickis. The power of the Fisher permutation test in 2 by *k* tables. *Commun Stat B*; 1984; 13: 433–448.
     x-tab/power/application.
298. Kryscio RJ; MH Meyers, SI Prusiner, HW Heise, and BW Christine. The space-time distribution of Hodgkin's disease in Connecticut, 1940–1969. *J Nat Cancer Inst*; 1973; 50: 1107–1110.
     Mantel/application.
299. Lachin JM. Properties of sample randomization in clinical trials. *Controlled Clinical Trials*; 1988; 9: 312–326.
     test/moments.
300. Lachin JN. Statistical properties of randomization in clinical trials. *Controlled Clinical Trials*; 1988; 9: 289–311.
     concept.
301. Lambert D. Influence functions for testing. *J Am Statist Assoc*; 1981; 76: 649–657.
     flaws and misuse/theory.
302. Lambert, D. Qualitative robustness of tests. *J Am Statist Assoc*; 1982; 77: 352–357.
     flaws and misuse/theory.
303. Lambert D. Robust two-sample permutation tests. *Annal of Statist*; 1985; 13: 606–625.
     test/robust.
304. Lambert. D; WJ Hall. Asymptotic lognormality of *p*-values. *Annal of Statist* 1982; 10: 44–64.
     theory.
305. Latscha R. Tests of significance in a $r \times r$ contingency table; extension of Finney's table. *Biometrika*: 1953; 40: 74–86.
     xtab/table.
306. Lee MLT. Tests of independence against LR dependence in ordered contingency tables. *Topics in Statistical Dependence*. HW Block, AR Sampson, TH Savits.

Hayward CA: IMS; 1990; 16: 351–357.
xtab.

307. Lefebvre M. Une application des methodes sequentielles aux tests de permuta-tions. *Canad J Statist*; 1982; 10: 173–180.
tests.

308. Lehmann EL. Consistancy and unbiasedness of certain nonparametric tests. *Annal Math Statist*; 1951; 22: 165–179.
theory/two-sample.

309. Lehmann EL. *Non-Parametrics: Statistical Methods Based on Ranks*. San Fran-cisco: Holden-Day; 1975.
p-dist.

310. Lehmann EL. *Testing Statistical Hypotheses*. New York: John Wiley & Sons; 1986.
theory/asymptotic/efficiency/power.

311. Lehmann EL; D'Abverra HJM. *Nonparametrics*. San Francisco: Holden-Day; 1975.
power.

312. Lehmann EL; Stein C. On the theory of some nonparametric hypotheses. *Annal Math Statist*; 1949; 20: 28–45.
power.

313. Leslie PH. A method of calculating the exact probabilities in 2×2 contingency tables with small marginal totals. *Biometrika*; 1955; 42: 522–523.
exact/xtab/algorithm.

314. Levin DA. The organization of genetic variability in Phlox drummondi. *Evolu-tion*; 1977; 31: 477–494.
Mantel/application.

315. Levin JM; LA Marascuilo, and LJ Hubert. Nonparametric randomization tests. JR Kratochwill, Editor. *Single Subject Research: Strategies for Evaluating Change*. New York: Academic Press; 1978: 167–196.
concept.

316. Lindsey JK. Likelihood analyses and test for binary data. *Appl Stat*; 1975; 241: 1–16.
conditional likelihood/design.

317. Livezey RE. Statistical analysis of general circulation model climate simula-tion: sensitivity and prediction experiments. *J of Atmospheric Sciences*; 1985; 42: 1139–1149.
review/application.

318. Livezey RE; W Chen. Statistical field significance and its determination by Monte Carlo techniques. *Monthly Weather Review*; 1983; 111: 46–59.
application.

319 Lock RH. A sequential approximation to a permutation test. *Commun Statist—Simul*; 1991; 20: 341–363.
algorithm.

320. Lorenz J; JH Eiler. Spawning habitat and characteristics of sockeye salmon in the Glacial Taker River, British Columbia and Alaska. *Transactions American Fisheries Society*; 1989; 18: 495–502.
application/choose.

321. Louis EJ; ER Dempster. An exact test for Hardy-Weinberg and multiple alleles. *Biometrics*; 1987; 43: 805–811.
misuse/model/*p*-dist/xtab.

322. Mackay DA; RE Jones. Leaf-shape and the host-finding behavior of two ovi-positing monophagous butterfly species. *Ecological Entomology*; 1989; 14: 423–431.
application.

323. Macuson R; E Nordbrock. A multivariate permutation test for the analysis of arbitrarily censored survival data *Biometrical J*; 1981; 23: 461–465. multivariate/censored.

324. Madow WG. On the limiting distribution of estimates based on samples from finite universes. *Annal Math Statist*; 1948; 19: 534–545. clt.

325. Manly BFJ. Analysis of polymorphic variation in different types of habitat. *Biometrics*; 1983; 39. *p*-dist/application.

326. Manly BFJ. The comparison and scaling of student assessment marks in several subjects. *Appl Statist*; 1988; 37: 385–395. choose/application.

327. Manly BFJ. *Randomization and Monte Carlo Methods in Biology*. London: Chapman and Hall; 1991. methods.

328. Mann HB. Nonparametric tests against trend. *Econometrica*; 1945; 13: 245–259. *p*-dist.

329. Mann RC; REJr Hand. The randomization test applied to flow cytometric histograms. *Computer Programs in Biomedicine*; 1983; 17: 95–100. application.

330. Mantel N. The detection of disease clustering and a generalized regression approach. *Cancer Research*; 1967; 27: 209–220. application/clusters/*p*-dist.

331. Mantel N. Re: "Clustering of disease in population units: an exact test and its asymptotic version." *Amer J Epidemiol*; 1983; 118: 628–629. choice/xtab/clustering/misuse/asymptotic.

332. Mantel N; JC Bailar. A class of permutational and multinomial tests arising in epidemiological research. *Biometrics*; 1970; 26: 687–700. application.

333. Mantel N; RS Valand. A technique of nonparametric multivariate analysis. *Biometrics*; 1970; 26: 547–558. application/*U*-statistics/multivariate.

334. Marascuilo LA; M McSweeny. *Nonparametric and Distribution-Free Methods for the Social Sciences*. Monterey CA: Brooks/ Cole; 1977. concept/review.

335. Marcus LF. Measurement of selection using distance statistics in prehistoric orang-utan pongo pygamous palaeosumativens. *Evolution*; 1969; 23: 301. application.

336. Maritz JS. *Distribution Free Statistical Methods*. London: Chapman and Hall; 1981. confidence intervals.

337. Marriott FHC. Barnard's Monte Carlo tests: How many simulations? *Appl Statist*; 1979; 28: 75–77. algorithm/Monte Carlo.

338. Marshall-Olds T. Analysis of local variation in plant size. *Ecology*; 1987; 68: 82–87. review/application.

339. Martin RL. On the design of experiments under spatial correlation. *Biometrika*; 1986; 73: 247–277. *p*-dist/design.

340. Martin-Lof P. Exact tests, confidence regions and estimates. Barndorff–Nielsen O, Blasild P, and Schow G. Proceeding of the Conference of Foundational Questions in Statistical Inference. Aarhus: Institute of Mathematics, University of Aarhus; 1974; 1: 121–138. concept.

341. McCarthy MD. On the application of the z-test to randomized blocks. *Annal Math Statist*; 1937; 10: 337–359.
     design.
342. McKinney PW; MJ Young, A Hartz, and M Bi-Fong Lee. The inexact use of Fisher's exact test in six major medical journals. *JAMA*; 1989; 261: 3430–3433.
     exact test/misuse/tests.
343. McLeod RS; DW Taylor, A Cohen, and JB Cullen. Single patient randomized clinical trials; its use in determining optimal treatment for patients with inflammation of a Kock continent ilestomy reservoir. *Lancet*; 1986; 29: 726–728.
     application, single-case.
344. Mead, R. A test for spatial pattern at several scales using data from a grid of contiguous quadrats. *Biometrics*; 1974; 30: 295–307.
     patterns.
345. Meagher TR; DS Burdick. The use of nearest neighbor frequency analysis in studies of association. *Ecology*; 1980; 61: 1253–1255.
     application.
346. Mehta CR; NR Patel, and LJ Wei. Computing exact permutational distributions with restricted randomization designs. *Biometrika*; 1988; 75: 295–302.
     algorithm/restricted/designs.
347. Mehta CR; NR Patel, and AA Tsiatis. Exact significance testing to establish treatment equivalence for ordered categorical data. *Biometrics*; 1984; 40: 819–825.
     algorithm/xtab.
348. Mehta CR; NR Patel, and P Senchaudhuri. Importance sampling for estimating exact probabilities in permutational inference. *J Am Statist Assoc*; 1988; 83: 999–1005.
     algorithm.
349. Mehta CR; NR Patel, and R Gray. On computing an exact confidence interval for the common odds ratio in several 2×2 contingency tables. *J Am Statist Assoc*; 1985; 80: 969–973.
     xtab/confidence/algorithm.
350. Melia KF; CL Ehlers. Signal detection analysis of ethanol effects on a complex conditional discrimination. *Pharm Biochem Behavior*; 33; 1989: 581–584.
     application/misuse.
351. Merrington M; CC Spicer. Acute leukemia in New England. *Brit J Preventive and Soc Med*; 1969; 23: 124–127.
     Mantel/application.
352. Mielke PW. Clarification and appropriate inferences for Mantel and Valand's nonparametric multivariate analysis technique. *Biometrics*; 1978; 34: 277–282.
     finite population/multi-response.
353. Mielke PWJr. Geometric concerns pertaining to applications of statistical tests in the atmospheric sciences. *J Atmospheric Sci*; 1985; 42: 1209–1212.
     concept/application.
354. Mielke PWJr. Meterological applications of permutation techniques based on distance functions. Krishnaiah PR and Sen PK, editors. *Handbook of Statistics*. Amsterdam: North-Holland; 1984; 4: 813–830.
     applic.
355. Mielke PWJr. Non-metric statistical analysis: Some metric alternatives. *J Statist Plan Infer*; 1986; 13: 377–387.
     concept/multivariate/cyclic data.
356. Mielke PWJr. On asymptotic nonnormality of null distributions of MRPP statistics. *Commun Statist A*; 1979; 8: 1541–1550.
     multivariate/quadratic assignment/MRPP/asymptotic.
357. Mielke PWJr. Some parametric, nonparametric and permutation inference pro-

cedures resulting from weather modification experiments. *Commun Statist A*; 1979; 8: 1083–1096.
multivariate/*k*-sample.

358. Mielke PWJr; KJ Berry, and GW Brier. Application of multiresponse permutation procedures for examining seasonal changes in monthly mean sea-level pressure patterns. *Monthly Weather Rev*; 1981; 109: 120–126.
application.

359. Mielke PW; KJ Berry. Asymptotic clarifications, generalizations, and concerns regarding an extended class of matched pairs tests based on powers of ranks. *Psychometrika*; 1985; 48: 483–485.
matched-pairs/choosing/asymptotic/robust/concept/Wilcoxon.

360. Mielke PWJr. KJ Berry, PJ Brockwell, and JS Williams. A class of nonparametric tests based on multiresponse permutation procedures. *Biometrika*; 1981; 68: 720–724.
asymptotic.

361. Mielke PWJr; KJ Berry, and J Medina. Climax I and II: distortion resistant residual analysis. *J Appl Meterol*; 1982; 21: 788–792.
application/misuse.

362. Mielke PWJr; KJ Berry. An extended class of matched pairs tests based on powers of ranks. *Psychometrika*; 1976; 41: 84–100.
matched-pairs.

363. Mielke PWJr; KJ Berry. An extended class of permutation techniques for matched pairs. *Commun Statist—Theory and Methodology*; 1982; 11: 1197–1207.
tests/matched-pairs.

364. Mielke PWJr; KJ Berry, and ES Johnson. Multiresponse permutation procedures for a priori classifications. *Commun Statist*; 1976; A5(14): 1409–1424.
classification.

365. Mielke PWJr; KJ Berry. Non-asymptotic inferences based on the chi-square statistic for $r \times c$ contingency tables. *J Statist Plan Infer*; 1985; 12: 41–45.
algorithm/*p*-dist/Pearson type III/xtab.

366. Mielke PWJr; HK Iyer. Permutation techniques for analyzing multi-response data from randomized block experiments. *Commun Statist A*; 1982; 11: 1427–1437.
design/matched-pairs/multivariate.

367. Mielke PWJr; PK Sen. On asymptotic non-normal null distributions for locally most powerful rank tests statistics. *Commun Statist A*; 1981; 10: 1079–1094.
asymptotic.

368. Miller AJ; DE Shaw, LG Veitch, and EJ Smith. Analyzing the results of a cloud-seeding experiment in Tasmania. *Commun Statist A*; 1979; 8: 1017–1047.
application/residuals/choice.

369. Miller RG. *Simultaneous Statistical Inference*. New York: Springer-Verlag; 1956 (2nd Edition).
design/*p*-dist/simultaneous.

370. Mitchell-Olds T. Analysis of local variation in plant size. *Ecology*; 1987; 68: 82–87.
review.

371. Mitchell-Olds T. Quantitative genetics of survival and growth in Impatiens capensis. *Evolution*; 1986; 40.
application.

372. Mitra SK. On the *F*-test in the intrablock analysis of a balanced incomplete block design. *Sankhya*; 1961; 22: 279–84. design/moments.

373. Motoo M. On the Hoeffding's combinatorial central limit theorem. *Annal Inst Statist Math*; 1957; 8: 145–154.
clt.

374. Mueller LD; L Altenberg. Statistical inference on measures of niche overlap. Ecology; 1985; 66: 1204–1210.
   application.

375. Mukhopadhyay I. Nonparametric tests for multiple regression under permutation symmetry. *Calcutta Statist Assoc Bull*; 1989; 33: 93–114.
   tests.

376. Murphy BP. Comparison of some two-sample tests by means of simulation. *Commun Statist—Simulation*; 1976; B5: 23–32.
   power/simulation.

377. Nguyen TT. A generalization of Fisher s exact test in $p \times q$ contingency tables using more concordant relations. *Commun Statist B*; 1985; 14: 633–645.
   xtab/choice.

378. Nicholson TAJ. A method for optimizing permutation probabilities and its industrial applications. in *PJA Welsh Ed. Combinatorial Mathematics and its Applications*. NY: Academic Press; 1971: 201–217.
   algorithm.

379. Noether GE. Asymptotic properties of the Wald-Wolfowitz test of randomness. *Annal Math Statist*; 1950; 21: 231–246.
   asymptotic/trend/independence.

380. Noether, GE. Distribution-free confidence intervals. *Statistica Neerlandica*; 1978; 32: 104–122.
   confidence-interval.

381. Noether GE. On a theorem by Wald and Wolfowitz. *Annal Math Statist*; 1949; 20.
   clt.

382. Noreen E. *Computer-Intensive Methods for Testing Hypotheses*. New York: John Wiley & Sons; 1989.
   bootstrap vs/algorithm/power.

383. O'Reilly FJ; PWJr Mielke. Asymptotic normality of MRPP statistics from invariance principles of U-statistics. *Commun Statist A*; 1980; 9: 629–637.
   MRPP/asymptotic.

384. O'Sullivan F; P Whitney, MM Hinshelwood, and ER Hauser. Analysis of repeated measurement experiments in endocrinology. *J Anim Science*; 1989; 59: 1070–1079.
   repeated measurements/application.

385. Oden A; H Wedel. Arguments for Fisher's permutation test. *Annal Statist* 1975; 3: 518–520.
   Robustness.

386. Oden NL. Allocation of effort in Monte Carlo simulations for power of permutation tests. *J Am Statist Assoc*; 1991; 86: 1074–1076.
   power/Monte Carlo.

387. Ogawa J. Effect of randomization on the analysis of a randomized block design. *Annal Inst Stat Math Tokyo*; 1961; 13: 105–117.
   design/p-dist.

388. Ogawa J. Exact and approximate sampling distribution of the F-statistic under the randomization procedure. in *A Modern Course on Statistical Distributions in Scientific Work*. GP Patil, S Kotz, and JK Ord Eds. Dordret-Holland: Reidel Publishing Company; 1975.
   p-dist.

389. Ogawa J. On the null distribution of the F-statistic in a randomized block under the Neyman model. *Annals Math Statist*; 1963. 34: 1558.
   design.

390. Ogawa J. *Statistical Theory of the Analysis of Experimental Designs*. New York: Marcel Dekker; 1974.
   design.

391. Ogbonmwan E; A Wynn. Resampling generalized likelihoods. *Statistical Decision Theory and Related Topics*. Gupta SS and JO Berger, Eds. New York: Springer Verlag; 1988; 1: 133–147.
    concept/resampllng.
392. Oja Hannu. On permutation tests in multiple regression and analysis of covariance problems. *Austral J Statist*; 1987; 29: 91–100.
    tests.
393. Pallini A; F Pesarin. A class of combinations of dependent tests by bootstrap and permutations procedures (abstract only). *IMS Bulletin*; 1990; 19: 574–575.
    combination of tests.
394. Passing H. Exact simultaneous comparisons with controls in an $r \times c$ contingency table. *Biometrical J*; 1984; 26: 643–654.
    cross-tab/simultaneous.
395. Patefield WM. Exact tests for trends in ordered contingency tables. *Appl Statist*; 1982; 31: 32–43.
    xtab.
396. Patil CHK. Cochran's Q test: exact distribution. *J Am Statist Assoc*; 1975; 70: 186–189.
    contingency.
397. Pearson ES. Some aspects of the problem of randomization. *Biometrika*; 1937; 29: 53–64.
    concept/choice of test/alternative.
398. Pecaric JE; F Proschan, and YL Tong. *Convex Functions, Partial Orderings, and Statistical Applications*. Boston: Academic Press; 1992.
    theory/likelihood.
399. Peritz E. Exact tests for matched pairs: studies with covariates. *Commun Statist A*; 1982; 11: 2157–2167 (errata 12: 1209–1210).
    matched-pairs/covariate.
400. Peritz E. Modified Mantel–Haenszel procedures for matched pairs. *Commun Statist A*; 1985; 14: 2263–2285.
    matched pairs/logistic/covariates.
401. Peto R; J Peto. Asymptotically efficient rank invariant test procedures. *J Roy Statist Soc A*; 1972; 135: 185–206.
    survival/censor/power.
402. Petrondas DA; RK Gabriel. Multiple comparisons by rerandomization tests. *J Am Statist Assoc*; 1983; 78: 949–957.
    multiple comparisons.
403. Picard R. Randomization and design. *RA Fisher, An Appreciation*. SE Fienberg and DV Hinckley, Editors. New York: Springer-Verlag; 1980: 208–213.
    test.
404. Pike MC; PG Smith. A case-control approach to examine disease for evidence of contagion including diseases with long latent periods. *Biometrics*; 1974; 30: 263–279.
    cluster/covariate/case-control/restricted.
405. Pitman EJG. Significance tests which may be applied to samples from any population. *Roy Statist Soc Suppl*; 1937; 4: 11–130, 225–232.
    concept/tests.
406. Pitman EJG. Significance tests which may be applied to samples from any population. Part III. The analysis of variance test. *Biometrika*; 1938; 29: 322–335.
    tests.
407. Plackett RL. *Analysis of Categorical Data*. London: Griffin; 1974.
    exact/reference set.

408. Plackett RL. Analysis of permutations. *Applied Statistics*; 1975; 24: 163–171.
logistic models/application.

409. Plackett RL. Random permutations. *J Roy Stat Soc B*; 1968; 30: 517–534.
algorithm.

410. Pollard E; KH Lakhand, and P Rothrey. The detection of density dependence from a series of annual censuses. *Ecology*; 1987; 68: 2046–2055.
application.

411. Prager MH; JM Hoenig. Superposed epoch analysis: A randomization test of environmental effects on recruitment with application to chub mackrel. *Transac Am Fisheries Soc*; 1989; 18: 608–619.
application/misuse.

412. Priesendorfer RW; TP Barnett. Numerical model/reality intercomparison tests using small-sample statistics. *J of Atmospheric Sci*; 1983; 40: 1884–1896.
p-dist/choosing/application.

413. Puri M; PK Sen. *Non-parametric Methods in General Linear Models*. New York: John Wiley; 1985.
multivariate/ranks/design.

414. Puri ML; PK Sen. A class of rank order tests for a general linear hypothesis. *Annal Math Statist*; 1969; 40: 1325–1343.
multivariate.

415. Puri ML; PK Sen. *Nonparametric Techniques in Multivariate Analysis*. New York: John Wiley and Sons; 1971.
clt.

416. Puri ML; PK Sen. On a class of multivariate, multisample rank-order tests. *Sankyha Ser A*; 1966; 28: 353–376.
tests/multivariate.

417. Puri ML; HD Shane. Statistical inference in incomplete blocks design. *Nonparametric Techniques in Statistical Inference*. ML Puri, Ed. Cambridge: University Press; 1970: 131–155.
p-dist.

418. Putter J. Treatment of ties in some nonparametric tests. *Annal Math Statist*; 1955; 26: 368–386.
p-dist.

419. Pyhel N. Distribution free *r*-sample tests for the hypothesis of parallelism of response profiles. *Biometric J*; 1980; 22: 703–714.
k-sample/response curves.

420. Quinn, JF. On the statistical detection of cycles in extinctions in the marine fossil record. *Paleobiology*; 1987; 13: 465–478.
application/trend.

421. Randles RH; DA Wolfe. *Introduction to the Theory of Nonparametric Statistics*. New York: John Wiley and Sons; 1979.
review/robust.

422. Rao JNK; DR Bellhouse. Optimal estimation of a finite population mean under generalized random permutation models. *J Statist Plan and Infer*; 1978; 2: 125–141.
estimation.

423. Rao TJ. Some aspects of random permutation models in finite population sampling theory. *Metrika*; 84; 31: 25–32.
design.

424. Ray W. Logic for a rank test. *Behav Science*; 1966; 11: 405.
algorithm.

425. Raz J. Analysis of repeated measurements using nonparametric smoothing and randomization tests. *Biometrics*; 1989; 45: 851–871.
repeated measurements.

426. Raz J. Testing for no effect when estimating a smooth function by nonparametric regression: a randomization approach. *JASA*; 1990; 85: 132–138.
tests/dependence/*p*-dist.

427. Recchia M; M Recchetti. The simulated randomization test. *Computer Programs in Biomedicine*; 1982; 15: 111–116.
concept.

428. Rice WR. A new probability model for determining exact *p*-values for 2×2 contingency tables when comparing binomial proportions. *Biometrics*; 1988; 44: 1–14.
x-tab.

429. Ritland C; K Ritland. Variation of sex allocation among eight taxa of the Minimuls guttatus species complex (Scrophulariaceae). *Amer J Botany*; 1989; 76.
Application.

430. Roberson P; L Fisher. Lack of robustness in time-space disease clustering. *Commun Statist B: Simulation and Computing*; 1986; 12: 11–22.
clusters/misuse.

431. Robinson J. Approximations to some test statistics for permutation tests in a completely randomized design. *Austral J Statist*; 1983; 25: 358–369.
asymptotic/design.

432. Robinson J. An asymptotic expansion for samples from a finite population. *Annal Statist*; 1978; 6: 1005–1011.
asymptotic.

433. Robinson J. An asymptotic expansion for permutation tests with several samples. *Annal Statist*; 1980; 8: 851–864.
asymptotic/*k*-sample.

434. Robinson J. A converse to a combinatorial central limit theorem. *Annal Math Statist*; 1972; 43: 2055–2057.
asymptotic/theory.

435. Robinson J. Large deviation probabilities for samples from a finite population. *Annal Probability*; 1977; 5: 913–925.
theory/asymptotic.

436. Robinson J. The large-sample power of permutation tests for randomization models. *Annal Statist*; 1973; 1: 291–296.
power/asymptotic.

437. Robinson, J. Nonparametric confidence intervals in regression: The bootstrap and randomization methods. *New Perspectives in Theoretical and Applied Statistics*. M Puri, JP Vilaplana, and W Wertz, Eds. New York: John Wiley & Sons; 1987: 243–256.
confidence/bootstrap.

438. Robinson J. On the test for additivity in a randomized block design. *J Am Statist Assoc*; 1975; 70: 184–194.
p-dist/design/asymptotic.

439. Romano JP. Bootstrap and randomization tests of some nonparametric hypotheses. *Annal Statist*; 1989; 17: 141–159.
efficiency.

440. Romano JP. On the behavior of randomization tests without a group invariance assumption. *J Am Statist Assoc*; 1990; 85: 686–692.
robust/misuse/asymptotic.

441. Romesburg HC. Exploring, confirming and randomization techniques. *Computers and Geosciences*; 1985; 11: 19–37.
multivariate/concept/program/discrim anal.

442. Rosen B. Limit theorems for sampling from a finite population. *Ark Mat*; 1965; 5: 383–424.
limit/finite/theory.

443. Rosenbaum PR. Conditional permutation tests and the propensity score in observational studies. *JASA*; 1984; 79: 565–574.
tests.

444. Rosenbaum PR. On permutation tests for hidden biases in observational studies: an application of Holley's inequality to the Savage lattice. *Annal Statist*; 1989; 17: 643–653.
p-dist.

445. Rosenbaum PR. Permutation tests for matched pairs with adjustments for covariates. *Appl Statist*; 1988; 37: 401–411.
covariates.

446. Rosenbaum PR. Sensitivity analysis for certain permutation tests in matched observational studies. *Biometrika*; 1987; 74: 13–26.
p-dist/power.

447. Rosenbaum PR. Sensitivity analysis for matching with multiple controls. *Biometrika*; 1988; 75: 577–581.
restricted.

448. Rosenbaum PR. Sensitivity analysis for matched observational studies with many ordered treatments. *Scand J Statist*; 1989; 16: 227–236.
matching/observational studies.

449. Rosenbaum PR. Sensitivity analysis for matched case-control studies. *Biometrics*; 1991; 47: 87–100.
matched pairs/observational.

450. Rosenbaum PR; AM Krieger. Sensitivity analysis of two-sample permutation inferences in observational studies. *J Am Statist Assoc*; 1990; 85: 493–498.

451. Royaltey HH; E Astrachen, and RR Sokal. Tests for patterns in geographic variation. *Geographic Analys*; 1975; 7: 369–395.
application.

452. Rubin DB. Bayesian inference for causal effects: the role of randomization. *Annal Statist*; 1978; 6: 34–58.
theory.

453. Ryman N; C Reuterwall, K Nygren, and T Nygren. Genetic variation and differentiation in Scandiavian moose (Alces): Are large mammals monomorphic? *Evolution*; 1980; 34: 1037–1049.
application.

454. Salsburg DS. *The Use of Restricted Significance Tests in Clinical Trials*. New York: Springer-Verlag; 1992.
application/restricted/clinical trials.

455. Scheffe H. *Analysis of Variance*. New York: John Wiley and Sons; 1959.
design.

456. Scheffe H. Statistical inference in the non-parametric case. Annals Math Statist; 1943; 14: 305–332.
concept.

457. Schemper M. A generalization of the intraclass tau correlation for tied and censored data. *Biometrical J*; 1984; 26: 609–617.
xtab/censored.

458. Schemper M. A survey of permutation tests for censored survival data. *Commun Stat A*; 1984; 13: 433–448.
power.

459. Schrage C. Evaluation of permutation tests by means of normal approximation or Monte Carlo methods. *Comput Statist Quart*; 1984; 1: 325–332.
approximation/Monte Carlo.

460. Schulman RS. Ordinal data; an alternative distribution. *Psychometrika*; 1979; 44: 3–20.
conditional *p*-dist/rank test/trend.

461. Schultz JR; L Hubert. A nonparametric test for the correspondence between two proximity matrices. *J Educ Statist*; 1976; 1: 59–67.
     Mantel/concept.
462. Selander RK; DW Kaufman. Genetic structure of populations of the brown snail (Helix aspersa). I: Microgeographic variation. *Evolution*; 1975; 29: 385–401.
     Mantel/application.
463. Sen PK. Nonparametric tests for multivariate interchangeability. Part 1: Problems of location and scale in bivariate distributions. *Sankhya A*; 1967; 29: 351–372.
     multivariate.
464. Sen PK. Nonparametric tests for multivariate interchangeability. Part 2: The problem of MANOVA in two-way layouts. *Sankhya*; 1969; 31.
     multivariate.
465. Sen PK. On permutational central limit theorems for general multivariate linear statistics. *Sankhya A*; 1983; 45: 141–149.
     multivariate/clt.
466. Sen PK. On some permutation tests based on U-statistics. *Bull Calcutta Stat Assoc*; 1965; 14: 106–126.
     U statistics/tests.
467. Sen PK. On some multisample permutation tests based on a class of U-statistic. *J Am Statist Assoc*; 1967; 62: 1201–1213.
     U-statistic.
468. Sen PK; ML Puri. On the theory of rank order tests for location in the multivariate one sample problem. *Annal Math Statist*; 1967; 38: 1216–1228.
     multivariate.
469. Servy EC; PK Sen. Missing variables in multi-sample rank permutation tests for MANOVA and MANCOVA. *Sankhya A*; 1987; 49: 78–95.
     efficiency/multivariate/design/ranks.
470. Shane HD; ML Puri. Rank order tests for multivariate paired comparisons. *Annal Math Statist*; 1969; 40: 2101–2117.
     multivariate/matched-pairs.
471. Shapiro CP; LJ Hubert. Asymptotic normality of permutation probabilities derived from the weighted sums of bivariate functions. *Annal Statist*; 1979; 7: 788–794.
     bivariate/asymptotic.
472. Shen CD; D Quade. A randomization test for a three-period three-treatment crossover experiment. *Commun Statist B*; 12. missing/design/multi-period/application.
473. Shorack G. Testing and estimating ratios of scale parameters. *J Am Statist Assoc*; 1969; 64: 999–1013.
     asymptotic approximation/test.
474. Shuster JJ; JM Boyett. Nonparametric multiple comparison procedures. *J Am Statist Assoc*; 1979; 74: 379–382.
     multiple comparisons.
475. Siegel S. *Practical Nonparametric Statistics*. New York: Wiley; 1956.
     test.
476. Siemiatycki J. Mantel's space-time clustering statistic: computing higher moments and a comparison of various data transforms. *J Statist Comput Simul*; 1978; 7: 13–31.
     approximatlon/cluster.
477. Siemiatycki J; AD McDonald. Neural tube defects in Quebec: A search for evidence of clustering in time and space. Brit *J Prev Soc Med*, 1972; 26: 10–14.
     application.
478. Silvey SD. Asymptotic distributions of statistics arising in certain nonparametric

tests. *Proc Glascow Math Assoc*; 1956; 2: 47–51.
asymptotic/p-dist/variance.

479. Silvey SD. Equivalence of asymptotic distributions arising under randomization and normal theories. *Proc Glascow Math Assoc*; 1954; 1: 139–147.
asymptotic.

480. Simon R. Restricted randomization designs in clinical trials. *Biometrics*; 1979; 35: 503–512.
clinical trials.

481. Smith PG; MC Pike. Generalization of two tests for the detection of household aggregation of disease. *Biometrics*; 1976; 32: 817–828.
application/p-dist/clustering.

482. Smith RL. Sequential treatment allocation using biased coin designs. *J Roy Statist Soc B*; 1984; 46: 519–543.
inference/concept/p-dist.

483. Smythe RT. Conditional inference for restricted randomization designs. *Annal Math Statist*; 1988; 16: 1155–1161.
restricted.

484. Smythe RT; LJ Wei. Significance tests with restricted randomization design. *Biometrika*; 1983; 70: 496–500.
p-dist/restricted.

485. Sokal RR. Testing statistical significance in geographical variation patterns. *Systematic Zoology*; 1979; 28: 227–232.
Mantel/application.

486. Sokal RR; FJ Rohlf. *Biometry*. San Francisco: Freeman; 1981.
application.

487. Solow AR. A randomization test for independence of animal locations. *Ecology*; 1989; 70.
application.

488. Solow AR. A randomization test for misclassification problems in discriminatory analysis. *Ecology*; 1990; 71: 2379–2382.
discriminatory analysis.

489. Soms AP. Permutation tests for k-sample binomial data with comparisons of exact and approximate P-levels. *Commun Statist A*; 1985; 14.
binomial/test.

490. Spino C; M Pagano. Efficient calculation of the permutation distribution of trimmed means. *J Am Statist Assoc*; 1991; 86: 729–737.
algorithm/asymptotic/outliers/matched pairs.

491. Steyn HS; RH Stumpf. Exact distributions associated with an $h \times k$ contingency table. *S African Stat J*; 1984; 18: 135–159.
xtab.

492. Still AW; AP White. The approximate randomization test as an alternative to the F-test in the analysis of variance. British *J Math Stat Psych*; 1981; 34: 243–252.
concept/robust/review.

493. Storer BE; C Kim. Exact properties of some exact test statistics for comparing two binomial populations. *J Am Statist Assoc*; 1990; 85: 146–155.
xtab.

494. Stucky W; J Vollmar. Ein verfahren zur exakten awwertung von $r \times c$-haufigeekeitstatein. *Biom Zeit*; 1975; 17: 147–162.
xtab.

495. Suissa S; JJ Shuster. Are uniformly most powerful unbiased tests really best? *Am Statistician*; 1984; 38: 204–206.
xtab/concept/misuse.

496. Suissa S; J Shuster. Exact unconditional sample sizes for the 2×2 binomial

trial. *J Roy Statist Soc A*; 1985; 148: 317–327.
xtab/power.

497. Takaeuchi K. Asymptotically efficient tests for location: nonparametric and asymptotically nonparametric. in *Nonparametric Techniques in Statistical Inference*. ML Puri, Ed. Cambridge: University Press; 1970: 131–155.
robust.

498. Tardif S. On the almost sure convergence of the permutation distribution for aligned rank test statistics in randomized block designs. *Annal Statist*; 1981; 9: 190–93.
asymptotic/rank/design.

499. Tocher KD. Extension of the Neyman-Pearson theory of tests of discontinuous variates. *Biometrika*; 1950; 37: 1301–1444.
xtab/inference.

500. Tracy DS; KA Khan. Comparison of some MRPP and standard rank tests for two unequal samples. *Commun Statist B*; 1989; 18: 729–756.
MRPP/power.

501. Tracy DS; KA Khan. Comparison of some MRPP and standard rank tests for three equal sized samples. *Commun Statist B*; 1990; 19: 315–333.
MRPP/power.

502. Tracy DS; IH Tajuddin. Empirical power comparisons of two MRPP rank tests. *Commun Statist A*; 1986; 15: 551–570.
MRPP/power.

503. Tracy DS; IH Tajuddin. Extended moment results for improved inferences based on MRPP. *Commun Statist A*; 1985; 14: 1485–1496.
MRPP.

504. Tritchler D. On inverting permutation tests. *J Am Statist Assoc*; 1984; 79: 200–207.
confidence intervals.

505. Tsutakawa RK; SL Yang. Permutation tests applied to antibiotic drug resistance. *JASA*; 1974; 69: 87–92.
application.

506. Tukey JW. Dyaclic ANOVA, an analysis of variance for vectors. *Human Biology*; 1949; 21: 65–110.

507. Tukey JW. Improving crucial randomized experiments—especially in weather modification—by double randomization and rank combination. Proceedings of the Berkeley Conference in Honor of J Neyman and J Kiefer, L LeCam, RA Olshen, CS Cheng, Editors. Hayward, CA: Institute of Mathematical Statistics; 1985; 1: 79–108.

508. Tukey JW; DR Brillinger, and LV Jones. *Management of Weather Resources*: Vol II: *The role of statistics in weather resources management*. Washington DC: Department of Commerce, US Government Printing Office; 1978.
power/concept/application.

509. Turnbull BW; EJ Iwano, WS Burnett, HL Howe, and LC Clark. Monitoring for clusters of disease: applications to leukemia incidence in upstate New York. *Am J Epidem*; 1990; 132: S136–143.
cluster/application.

510. Upton GJG. A comparison of alternative tests for the 2 × 2 comparative trial. *J Roy Statist Soc A*; 1982; 145: 86–105.
xtab.

511. Upton GJG; D Brook. Determination of the optimum position on a ballot paper. *Appl Stat*; 1975; 24: 279–287.
algorithm.

512. Vadiveloo, J. On the theory of modified randomization tests for nonparametric hypothesis. *Commun Statist—Theory and Methods*; 1983; 12: 1581–1598.
power/Monte Carlo.

513. van den Brink WP; SGJ van den Brink. A modified approximate permutation test procedure. *Comp Sci Quart*; 1990; 3: 241–247.
     test/algorithm/multistage.
514. van-Putten B. On the construction of multivariate permutation tests in the multivariate two-sample case. *Statist Neerlandica*; 1987; 41: 191–201.
     multivariate.
515. Vecchia DF; HK Iyer. Moments of the quartic assignment statistic with an application to multiple regression. *Common Statist—Theor and Meth*; 1991; 20: 3253–3269.
     cluster/multiple/Pearson.
516. Vecchia DF; Iyer HK. Exact distribution-free tests for equality of several linear models. *Commun Stat A*; 1989; 18: 2467–2488.
     MRPP/concept/review/cluster.
517. Wald A; J Wolfowitz. An exact test for randomness in the nonparametric case based on serial correlation. *Annal Math Statist*; 1943; 14: 378–388.
     time-series.
518. Wald A; J Wolfowitz. Statistical tests based on permutations of the observations. *Annal Math Statist*; 1944; 15: 358–372.
     clt/p-dist/tests/concept.
519. Wampold BE; MJ Furlong. Randomization tests in single-subject designs: illustrative examples. *J Behav Assess*; 1981; 3: 329–341.
     application.
520. Wei LJ. Exact two-sample permutation tests based on the randomized play-the-winner rule. *Biometrika*; 1988; 75: 603–605.
     restricted randomization.
521. Wei LJ; JM Lachin. Properties of urn-randomization in clinical trials. *Controlled Clinical Trials*; 1988; 9: 345–364.
     restricted randomization.
522. Wei LJ; RT Smythe, and RL Smith. K-treatment comparisons in clinical trials. *Annal Math Statist*; 1986; 14: 265–274.
     clinical trials/restricted.
523. Welch BL. On tests for homogenity. *Biometrika*; 1938; 30: 149–158.
     finite populations/concept/variance.
524. Welch BL. On the z-test in randomized blocks and Latin squares. *Biometrika*; 1937; 29: 21–52.
     concept/tests/p-dist/design.
525. Welch WJ. Construction of permutation tests. *J Am Statist Assoc*; 1990; 85: 693–698.
     review/theory/design.
526. Welch WJ. Rerandomizing the median in matched-pairs designs. *Biometrika*; 1987; 74: 609–614.
     robust/matched-pairs.
527. Welch WJ; LG Guitierrez. Robust permutation tests for matched pairs designs. *JASA*; 1988; 83: 450–461.
     robust/outliers.
528. Wellner JA. Permutation tests for directional data. *Annal Statist*; 1979; 7: 929–943.
     tests.
529. Westfall PH; SS Young. *Resampling-Based Multiple Testing*. New York: John Wiley & Sons; 1993.
530. Whaley FS. The equivalence of three individually derived permutation procedures for testing the homogenity of multidimensional samples. *Biometrics*; 1983; 39: 741–745.
     concept/multivariate.
531. White AP; AW Still. Monte Carlo analysis of variance. Proceedings of the 6th

Symposium in Computational Statistics. Havranek P, Z Sidak, and M Novak, Eds. Wien: Physica-Verlag; 1984.
design/robust/Monte Carlo.

532. Wilk MB. The randomization analysis of a generalized randomized block design. *Biometrika*, 1955; 42: 70–79.
designs.

533. Wilk MB; O Kempthorne. Nonadditivities in a Latin square design. *J Am Statist Assoc* 1957; 52: 218–236.
p-dist/design/average.

534. Wilk MB; O Kempthorne. Some aspects of the analysis of factorial experiments in a completely randomized design. *Annal Math Statist*; 1956; 27: 950–984.
p-dist.

535. Williams–Blangero S. Clan-structured migration and phenotypic differentiation in the Jirels of Nepal. *Hum Biol*; 1989; 61: 143–157.
spatial dispersion.

536. Witting, H. On the theory of nonparametric tests. In *Nonparametric Techniques in Statistical Inference*. ML Puri, Ed. Cambridge: University Press; 1970: 41–51.
groups/derivation/power.

537. Wong RKW; Chidambaram & Mielke PW. Applications of multi-response permutation procedures and median regression for covariate analyses of possible weather modification effects on hail responses. *Atmosphere-Ocean*; 1983; 21: 1–13.
MRPP/application/covariate.

538. Yanagimoto T; M Okamoto. Partial orderings for permutations and monotonicity of a rank correlation statistic. *Inst Stat Math Annal*; 1969; 21: 489–506.
power/theory/algorithm.

539. Yates F. Tests of significance for 2×2 contingency tables (with discussion). *J Roy Statist Soc A*; 1984; 147: 426–463.
xtab.

540. Young, A. Conditional data-based simulations. Some examples from geometric statistics. *Int Statist Rev*, 1986; 54: 1–13.
application/bootstrap.

541. Zelen M. The analysis of several 2×2 contingency tables. *Biometrika*; 1971; 58: 129–137.
concept/xtab/binomial/test.

542. Zerbe GO. Randomization analysis of the completely randomized design extended to growth and response curves. *J Am Statist Assoc*; 1979; 74: 215–221.
test/application/repeated measures.

543. Zerbe GO. Randomization analysis of randomized block design extended to growth and response curves. *Commun Statist A*; 1979; 8: 191–205.
design/repeated measures.

544. Zerbe GO; JR Murphy. On multiple comparisons in the randomization analysis of growth and response curves. *Biometrics*; 1986; 42: 795–804.
design/application.

545. Zerbe GO; SH Walker. A randomization test for comparison of groups of growth curves with different polynomial design matricies. *Biometrics*; 1977; 33: 653–657.
application/test.

546. Zimmerman GM; H Goetz, and PWJr Mielke. Use of an improved statistical method for group comparisons to study effects of prairie fire. *Ecology*; 1985; 66: 606–611.
application/MRPP.

BIBLIOGRAPHY PART 2:

Supporting

1. Berger JO; RW Wolpert. *The Likelihood Principle*. Institute of Mathematical Statistics Lecture Notes—Monograph Series. (1984) Heyward CA: IMS.
2. Bishop YMM; SE Fienberg, and PW Holland. *Discrete Multivariate Analysis: Theory and Practice*. (1975) Cambridge MA: MIT Press.
3. Box JF. *The Life of a Scientist*. (1978) New York: John Wiley and Sons.
4. Conover WJ; ME Johnson, and MM Johnson. Comparative study of tests for homogeneity of variances, with applications to the outer continental shelf bidding data. *Technometrics* 23, (1981) 351–361.
5. David HA. *Order Statistics*. (1970) New York: John Wiley and Sons.
6. Davis AW (1982). On the effects of moderate nonnormality on Roy's largest root test. *J Am Stat Assoc*; 77, 896–900.
7. Dodge Y. Editor, *Statistical Data Analysis Based on the L_1-norm and Related Methods*. (1987) Amsterdam: N Holland.
8. Efron B. Censored data and the bootstrap. *J Am Statist Assoc* 76, (1981) 312–319.
9. Efron B. Better bootstrap confidence intervals (with discussion). *J Am Statist Assoc*; (1987) 82, 171–200.
10. Fisher NI and Hall P. On bootstrap hypothesis testing. *Austral J Statist*; (1990) 32, 177–190.
11. Fix E; JLJr Hodges, and EL Lehmann. The restricted χ^2 test. In *Studies in Probability and Statistics Dedicated to Harold Cramer*. (1959) Stockholm: Almquist and Wiksell.
12. Gabriel KR. Ante-dependence analysis of an ordered set of variables. *Annal Math Statist*; (1962) 33, 201–212.
13. Gine E; J Zinn. Necessary conditions for a bootstrap of the mean. *Annal Statist*; (1989) 17, 684–691
14. Goodman L; W Kruskal. Measures of association for cross-classification. *J Am Statist Assoc* (1954) 49, 732–764.
15. Hall P; SR Wilson. Two guidelines for bootstrap hypothesis testing. *Biometrics*, (1991) 47, 757–762.
16. Hampel FR; EM Ronchetti, PJ Rousseeuw, and WA Stahel. *Robust Statistics: The Approach Based on Influence Functions*. (1986) New York: John Wiley and Sons.
17. Hasegawa M; H Kishino, and T Yano. Phylogentic inference from DNA sequence data. In *Statistical Theory and Data Analysis*. K Matusita, Ed. (1988) Amsterdam: North Holland.
18. Hodges JL; EL Lehmann. Testing the approximate validity of statistical hypothesis. *J Roy Statist Soc B*, 16, (1954) 261–268.

19. Hogg RV; RV Lenth. A review of some adaptive statistical techniques. *Comm Statist*, 13, (1984) 1551–1579.
20. Knight K. On the bootstrap of the sample mean in the infinite variance case. *Annals Statist*, 17, (1989) 1168–1173.
21. Lehmann E. Some concepts of dependence. *Annal Math Statist*, 37, (1966) 1137–1153.
22. Makridakis S; SC Wheelwright, and VE McGee. *Forecasting Methods and Applications*, (1983) New York: John Wiley and Sons.
23. Morrison DF. *Multivariate Statistical Methods*, (1990) New York: McGraw-Hill.
24. Smith R. Properties of biased coin designs in sequential clinical trials. *Annal Statist*, 12, (1984) 1018–1034.
25. Sampford MR; J Taylor. Censored observations in randomized block experiments. *J Roy Statist Soc B* 21(1), (1959) 214–237.
26. Stine RA. Estimating properties of autoregressive forecasts. *J Am Statist Assoc*, 82, (1987) 1072–1078.
27. Werner M; R Tolls, J Hultin, and J Mellecker. Sex and age dependence of serum calcium, inorganic phosphorous, total protein, and albumin in a large ambulatory population. In *Fifth Technical International Congress on Automation, Advances in Automated Analysis* 2: 59–65. (1970) Future Publishing Co., Mount Kisco, NY.

BIBLIOGRAPHY PART 3:

Computational Methods

1. Abramson M; WJ Moser. Arrays with fixed row and column sums. *Discrete Math*; 1973; 6: 1–14.
2. Agresti A; CR Mehta, and NR Patel. Exact inference for contingency tables with ordered categories. *Statist Assoc*; 1990; 85: 453–458.
3. AKl SG. A comparison of combination generation methods. ACM *Trans Math Software*; 1981; 7: 42–45.
4. Amana IA; GG Koch. A macro for multivariate randomization analysis of stratified sample data. *SAS Sugi*; 1980; 5: 134–144.
5. Arbuckle J; LS Astler. A program for Pitman's permutation test for differences in location. *Behav Res Meth and Instr*; 1975; 7: 381.
6. Baglivo J; D Olivier, and M Pagano. Methods for exact goodness-of-fit tests. *J Am Statist Assoc*; 1992; 87: 464–469.
7. Baglivo J; D Oliver, and M Pagano. Methods for the analysis of contingency Tables with large and small cell counts. *J Am Statist Assoc*; 1988; 83: 1006–1013.
8. Baker FB; RO Collier. Analysis of experimental designs by means of randomization, a Univac. 1103 program. *Behav Science*; 1961; 6: 369.
9. Baker RJ. Exact distributions derived from two-way tables. *Appl Statist*; 1977; 26: 199–206.
10. Balmer DW. Recursive enumeration of $r \times c$ tables for exact likelihood evaluation. AS 236. *Appl Statist*; 1988; 37: 290–301.
11. Bebbington AC. A simple method of drawing a sample without replacement. *Appl Statist*; 1975; 24: 136.
12. Bernard A; P Van Efferen. A generalization of the method of m rankings. Proc Kon Ned Akad Wefensch; 1953: A56.
13. Berry KJ. AS179 Enumeration of all permutations of multi-sets with fixed repetition numbers. *Appl Statist*; 1982; 31.
14. Besag J; P Clifford. Sequential Monte Carlo p-values *Biometrika*; 1991; 78: 301–304.
15. Bissell AF. Ordered random selection without replacement. *Appl Statist*; 1986; 35.
16. Bitner JR; G Ehrlich, and E Rheingold. Efficient generation of the reflected Gray Code and its applications. *Commun ACM*; 1976; 19: 517–521.
17. Booth JG; RW Butler. Random distributions and saddlepoint approximations in general linear models. *Biometrika*; 1990; 77: 787–796.
18. Boothroyd J. Algorithm 246. Gray code. *Commun ACM*; 1964; 7: 701.
19. Boothroyd J. Algorithm 29, Permutation of the elements of a vector. *Computer J*; 1967; 60: 311.

20. Boswell MT; SD Gore, GP Patel, and C Taillie. The art of computer generation of random variables. *Handbook of Statistics, 9. Computational Statistics.* CR Rao, Ed, Amsterdam: North Holland. 1993.

21. Boulton DM. Remarks on Algorithm 434. *Commun ACM*; 1974; 17: 326.

22. Boyet JM. Random $R \times C$ tables with given row and column totals (algorithm AS 144). *Appl Statist*; 1979; 28.

23. Bratley P. Algorithm 306, Permutations with repetitions. *Commun ACM*; 1967; 10: 450–451.

24. Chase PJ. Algorithm 382. Combinations of M out of N objects. *Commun ACM*; 1970a; 13: 368.

25. Chase PJ. Algorithm 383, Permutations of a set with repetitions. *Commun ACM*; 1970b; 13.

26. Dallal, GE. Pitman: A Fortran program for exact randomization tests. *Computers and Biomed Res*; 1988; 21: 9–15.

27. Daniels HE. Discussion of paper by GEP Box and SL Anderson. *J Roy Statist Soc B*; 1955; 17: 27–28.

28. Daniels HE. Discussion of paper by DR Cox. *J Roy Statist Soc B*; 1958; 20: 236–238.

29. Davison AC; DV Hinkley. Saddlepoint approximations in randomization methods. *Biometrika*; 1988; 75: 417–431.

30. De Cani J. An algorithm for bounding tail probabilities for two-variable exact tests. *Randomization*; 1979; 2: 23–4.

31. Dershowitz N. A simplified loop-free algorithm for generating permutations. *BIT*; 1975; 15: 158–164.

32. Durstenfield R. Random permutations. *Commun ACM*; 1964; 7: 420.

33. Ehrlich G. Algorithm 466. Four combinatorial algorithms. *Commun ACM*; 1973; 16: 690–691.

34. Feldman SE; E Kluger. Shortcut calculations to Fisher-Yates "exact tests". *Psychometrika*; 1963; 2: 289–291.

35. Fike CT. A permutation generation method. *Computer J*; 1975; 18: 21–22.

36. Fleishman AI. A program for calculating the exact probabilities along with explorations of m by n contingency tables. *Educ Psychol Measure*; 1977; 33: 798–803.

37. Gail M; N Mantel. Counting the number of $r \times c$ contingency tables with fixed marginals. *J Am Statist Assoc*; 1977; 72: 859–862.

38. Gentleman JF. Algorithm AS88. Generation of all nCr combinations by simulating nested Fortran DO loops. *Appl Statist*; 1975; 24: 374–376.

39. Goetgheluck P. Computing binomial coefficients. *Am Math Monthly*; 1987; 94: 360–365.

40. Green BF. A practical interactive program for randomization tests of location. *Am Statist*; 1977; 31: 37–39.

41. Gregory RJ. A Fortran computer program for the Fisher exact probability test. *Educ Psychol Measurement*; 1973; 33: 697–700.

42. Hancock TW. Remark on algorithm 434. *Commun ACM*; 1974; 18: 117–119.

43. Hayes JE. Fortran program for Fisher's exact test. *Behav Meth Instrum*; 7: 481.

44. Howell DC; LR Gordon. Computing the exact probability of an r by c contingency table with fixed marginal totals. *Behav Res Meth and Instr*; 1976; 8: 317.

45. Hull ID; R Peto. Alg AS35 Probabilities derived from finite populations. *Appl Statist*; 1971; 20: 99–105.

46. Ives FM. Permutation enumeration: four new permutation algorithms. *Commun ACM*; 1976; 19: 68–70.

47. Joe H. Extreme probabilities for contingency tables under row and column independence with applications to Fisher's exact test. *Commun Statist A*; 1988; 17: 3677–3685.

48. Joe H. An ordering of dependence for contingency tables. *Lin Alg Appl*; 1985; 70: 89–103.
49. Knott GD. A numbering system for permutations of combinations. *Commun ACM*; 1976; 19: 355–356.
50. Knuth DE. *The Art of Computer Programming, Vol 2 Semi-Numerical Algorithms*. Reading MA: Addison-Wesley; 1973.
51. Kreiner S. Analysis of multidimensional contingency tables by exact conditional frequencies; techniques and strategies. *Scand J Statist*; 1987; 14: 97–112.
52. Kurtzburg J. Algorithm 94. Combination. *Commun ACM*; 1962; 5: 344.
53. Lam CWH; LH Sotchen. Three new combination algorithms with the minimal-change property. *Commun ACM*; 1982; 25: 555–559.
54. Liu CH; DT Tang. Algorithm 452. Enumerating combinations of m out of n objects. *Commun ACM*; 1973; 16: 485.
55. Mackenzie G; M O'Flaherty. Direct simulation of nested Fortran DO loops. *Appl Statist*; 1982; 31: 71–74.
56. March DL. Exact probabilities for $R \times C$ contingency tables. *Commun ACM*; 1972; 15: 991–992.
57. Marsh NWA. Efficient generation of all binary patterns by Gray Code. *Appl Statist*; 1987; 36: 245–249.
58. Mehta CR; NR Patel. FEXACT: a Fortran subroutine for Fisher's exact test on unordered $r \times c$ contingency tables. *ACM Trans Math Software*; 1986; 12: 154–161.
59. Mehta CR; NR Patel. A hybrid algorithm for Fisher's exact test in unordered $r \times c$ contingency tables. *Commun Statist*; 1986; 15: 387–403.
60. Mehta CR; NR Patel. A network algorithm for the exact treatment of the $2 \times K$ contingency table. *Commun Statist B*; 1980; 9: 649–664.
61. Mehta CR; NR Patel. A network algorithm for performing Fisher's exact test in $r \times c$ contingency, tables. *J Am Statist Assoc*; 1983; 78: 427–434.
62. Minc H. Rearrangements. *Trans Am Math Soc*; 1971; 159: 497–504.
63. Nelson DE; GO Zerbe. A SAS/IML program to execute randomization of response curves with multiple comparisons. American Statistician; 1988; 42: 231–232.
64. Nigam AK; VK Gupta. A method of sampling with equal or unequal probabilities without replacement. *Appl Statist*; 1984; 33.
65. Nijenhuis A; HS Wilf. *Combinatorial Algorithms*. New York: Academic Press; 1978.
66. Oden NE. Allocation of effort in Monte Carlo simulation for power of permutation tests. *J Am Statist Assoc*; 1991; 86: 1074–1076.
67. Ord-Smith RJ. Generation of permutation sequences: Part 1. *Computer J*; 1970; 13: 152–155.
68. Ord-Smith RJ. Generation of permutation sequences: part 2. *Computer J*; 1971; 14: 136–139.
69. Pagano M; K Halvorsen. An algorithm for finding the exact significance levels of $r \times C$ contingency tables. *J Am Statist Assoc*; 1981; 76.
70. Pagano M; D Tritchler. On obtaining permutation distributions in polynomial time. *J Am Statist Assoc*; 1983; 78: 435–441.
71. Page ES. Note on generating random parameters. *Appl Statist*; 1967; 16: 273–274.
72. Page ES; LB Wilson. *An Introduction to Combinatorial Combinations*. Cambridge UK: Cambridge University Press; 1979.
73. Patefield WM. An efficient method of generating $r \times c$ tables with given row and column totals (algorithm AS 159). *Appl Statist*; 1981; 30: 91–97.
74. Payne WH; FM Ives. Combination generators. *ACM Tran Math Software*; 1979; 5: 163–172.

75. Rabinowitz; ML Berenson. A comparison of various methods of obtaining random order statistics for Monte Carlo computations. *Am Stat*; 1974; 28: 27–29.

76. Radlow R; EF Alf. An alternate marginal assessment of the accuracy of the chi-square test of goodness of fit. *J Am Statist Assoc*; 1975; 70: 811–813.

77. Robertson WH. Programming Fisher's exact method of comparing two percentages. *Technometrics*; 1960; 2: 103–107.

78. Robinson J. Saddlepoint approximations to permutation tests and confidence intervals. *J Roy Statist Soc, B*; 1982; 44: 91–101.

79. Rogers MS. A Philco 2000 program to exhibit distinguishably different permutations. Behav Science; 1964; 9: 289–299.

80. Rohl JS. Generating permutations by choosing. *Computer J*; 1978; 21: 302–305.

81. Romesburg HC; R Marshall, and TP Mauk. FITEST—A computer program for "exact chi-square" goodness of fit tests. *Computers and Geosciences*; 1981; 7: 457–458.

82. Roy MK. Evaluation of permutation algorithms. *Computer J*; 1978; 21: 296–301.

83. Sag TW. Algorithm 242. Permutation with a set of repetitions. *Commun ACM*; 1964; 7: 585.

84. Saunders IW. Enumeration of $r \times c$ tables with repeated row totals. Applied Statistics; 1984; 33: 340–352.

85. Shamos MI. Geometry and statistics: problems at the interface. In *Algorithms and Complexity: New Directions and Recent Results*. JF Traub Ed. New York: Academic Press; 1976: 251–279.

86. Soms AP. An algorithm for the discrete Fisher's permutation tests. *J Am Statist Assoc*; 1977; 72: 662–664.

87. Spino C; M Pagano. Efficient calculation of the permutation distribution of robust two-sample statistics. *Comput Statist Data Anal*; 1991; 12: 349–368.

88. Spino C; M Pagano. Efficient calculation of the permutation distribution of trimmed means. *J Am Statist Assoc*; 1991; 86: 729–737.

89. Streitberg B; R Rohmed. Exact distributions for permutation and rank tests: an introduction to some recently published algorithms. *Stat Software Newsletter*; 1986; 12: 10–17.

90. Streitberg B; Rohmel J. Exact distributions for rank- and permutation-tests in the general c-sample problem. *EDV in Medizin und Biologie*; 1987; 18: 12–19.

91. Sunter AB. List sequential sampling with equal or unequal probabilities without replacement. *Applied Statistics*; 1977; 26: 261–268.

92. Thomas D. Exact and asymptotic methods for the combination of 2×2 tables. *Computers Biomedical Res*; 1975; 8: 423–446.

93. Tritchler D. An algorithm for exact logistic regression. *J Am Statist Assoc*; 1984; 79: 709–711.

94. Tritchler DL; DT Pedrini. A computer program for Fisher's exact test. *Educ Psychol Meas*; 35: 717–720.

95. Verbeek A; PM Kroonenberg. A survey of algorithms for exact distribution of test statistics in $r \times c$ tables with fixed marginals. *Comput Statist Data Anal*; 1985; 3: 159–185.

96. Vitter JS. Faster methods for random sampling. *Commun ACM*; 1984; 27: 703–718.

97. Vollset SE; KF Hirji, and RM Elashoff. Fast computation of exact confidence limits for the common odds ratio in a series of 2×2 tables. *J Am Statist Assoc*; 1991; 86: 404–409.

98. Vollset SE; KF Hirji. A microcomputer program for exact and asymptotic analysis of several 2×2 tables. *Epidemiology*; 1991; 2: 217–220.

99. Walsh JE. An experimental method for obtaining random digits and permutations. *Sankhya*; 1957; 17: 355–360.
100. Wells MB. *Elements of Combinatorial Computing*. 1971. Oxford: Pergammon;
101. Wichmann, BA; Hill, ID. Algorithm AS 183: an efficient and portable pseudo-random number generator. *Appl Statist*; 1982; 31: 188–190.
102. Woodhill AD. Generation of permutation sequences. *Computer J*; 1977; 20: 346–349.
103. Wright T. A note on Pascal's triangle and simple random sampling. *College Math J*; 1984; 20: 59–66.
104. Zar JH. A fast efficient algorithm for the Fisher exact test. *Behav Res Meth and Instr*; 1987; 19: 413–414.
105. Zimmerman H. Exact calculations of permutation distributions for r dependent samples. *Biometrical J*; 1985; 27: 349–352.
106. Zimmerman H. Exact calculations for permutation distribution for r independent samples. *Biometrical J*; 1985; 27: 431–443.

BIBLIOGRAPHY PART 4:

Seminal Articles

1. Agresti A.; D Wackerly, and JM Boyett. Exact conditional tests for cross-classifications: approximations of attained significance levels. *Psychometrika*; 1979; 44: 75–83.
2. Albers W; PJ Bickel, and WR Van Zwet. Asymptotic expansions for the power of distribution-free tests in the one-sample problem. *Annal Statist*; 1976; 4: 108–156.
3. Arnold HJ. Permutation support for multivariate techniques. *Biometrika*; 1964; 51: 65–70.
4. Baker FB; RO Collier. Analysis of experimental designs by means of randomization, a Univac 1103 program. Behav Sci; 1961; 6: 369–369.
5. Barton DE; FN David. Randomization basis for multivariate tests. *Bull Int Statist Inst*; 1961; 39: 455–467.
6. Basu D. Randomization analysis of experimental data: The Fisher randomization test. *J Am Statist Assoc*; 1980; 75: 575–582.
7. Bell CB; KA Doksum. Some new distribution free statistics. *Anal Math Statist*; 1965; 36: 203–214.
8. Bickel PM; WR Van Zwet. Asymptotic expansion for the power of distribution free tests in the two-sample problem. *Annal Statist*; 1978; 6: 987–1004 (corr 1170–1171).
9. Box GEP; SL Anderson. Permutation theory in the development of robust criteria and the study of departures from assumptions. *J Roy Statist Soc B*; 1955; 17: 1–34.
10. Boyett JM; JJ Shuster. Nonparametric one-sided tests in multivariate analysis with medical applications. *J Am Statist Assoc*; 1977; 72: 665–668..
11. Bradley JV. *Distribution Free Statistical Tests*. New Jersey: Prentice-Hall; 1968.
12. Bross IDJ. Taking a covariable into account. *J Am Statist Assoc*; 1964; 59: 725–736.
13. Dwass M. Modified randomization tests for non-parametric hypotheses. *Annal Math Statist*; 1957; 28: 181–187.
14. Fisher RA. Coefficient of racial likeness and the future of craniometry. *J Roy Anthrop Soc*; 1936; 66: 57–63.
15. Fisher, RA. *The Design of Experiments* 6th Ed. New York: Hafner; 1951.
16. Gabriel KR; CF Hsu. Evaluation of the power of rerandomization tests, with application to weather modification experiments. *J Am Statist Assoc*; 1983; 78: 766–775.
17. Good PI. Globally almost powerful tests for censored data. *Nonparametric Statistics*; 1992; 1: 253–262.
18. Hoeffding W. Combinatorial central limit theorem. *Annal Math Statist*; 1951; 22.

19. Kempthorne O; TE Doerfler. The behavior of some significance tests under experimental randomization. *Biometrika*; 1969; 56: 231–248.
20. Kempthorne O. *Design and Analysis of Experiments*. 1952. New York: John Wiley and Sons.
21. Lehmann EL; C Stein. On the theory of some nonparametric hypotheses. *Annal Math Statist*; 1949; 20: 28–45.
22. Mantel N. The detection of disease clustering and a generalized regression approach. *Cancer Research*; 1967; 27: 209–220.
23. Mehta CR; NR Patel. A network algorithm for the exact treatment of the $2 \times K$ contingency table. *Commun Statist B*; 1980; 9: 649–664.
24. Mielke PW; KJ Berry and ES Johnson. Multiresponse permutation procedures for a priori classifications. *Commun Statist*; 1976; A5(14): 1409–1424.
25. Oden A; H Wedel. Arguments for Fisher's permutation test. *Annal Statist*; 1975; 3: 518–520.
26. Ogawa J. Effect of randomization on the analysis of a randomized block design. *Annal Inst Stat Math Tokyo*; 1961; 13: 105–117.
27. Pearson ES. Some aspects of the problem of randomization. *Biometrika*; 1937; 29: 53–64.
28. Pitman EJG. Significance tests which may be applied to samples from any population. Part III: The analysis of variance test. *Biometrika*; 1938; 29: 322–335.
29. Pitman EJG. Significance tests which may be applied to samples from any population. *Roy Statist Soc Suppl*; 1937; 4: 119–130, 225–232.
30. Plackett RL. Random permutations. *J Roy Stat Soc B*; 1968; 30: 517–534.
31. Robinson J. A converse to a combinatorial central limit theorem. *Annal Math Statist*; 1972; 43: 2055–2057.
32. Rosenbaum, PR. Conditional permutation tests and the propensity score in observational studies. *JASA*; 1984; 79: 565–574.
33. Tukey JW; DR Brillinger, and LV Jones. *Management of Weather Resources. Vol II: The role of statistics in weather resources management*. Washington DC: Department of Commerce, US Government Printing Office; 1978.
34. Wald A; J Wolfowitz. Statistical tests based on permutations of the observations. *Annal Math Statist*; 1944; 15: 358–372.

Index

Springer Series in Statistics

(continued from p. ii)